From Trauma to Triumph

How Alternate Therapies Saved My Life and How They Can Save You

Rachie Jean Foster

First published by Ultimate World Publishing 2023
Copyright © 2023 Rachie Jean Foster

ISBN

Paperback: 978-1-922982-42-1
Ebook: 978-1-922982-43-8

Rachie Jean Foster has asserted her rights under the Copyright, Designs and Patents Act 1988 to be identified as the author of this work. The information in this book is based on the author's experiences and opinions. The publisher specifically disclaims responsibility for any adverse consequences which may result from use of the information contained herein. Permission to use information has been sought by the author. Any breaches will be rectified in further editions of the book.

All rights reserved. No part of this publication may be reproduced, stored in or introduced into a retrieval system, or transmitted in any form, or by any means (electronic, mechanical, photocopying, recording or otherwise) without the prior written permission of the author. Any person who does any unauthorised act in relation to this publication may be liable to criminal prosecution and civil claims for damages. Enquiries should be made through the publisher.

Cover design: Ultimate World Publishing
Layout and typesetting: Ultimate World Publishing
Editor: Rebecca Low

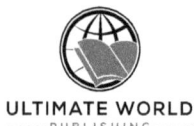

Ultimate World Publishing
Diamond Creek,
Victoria Australia 3089
www.writeabook.com.au

Dedication

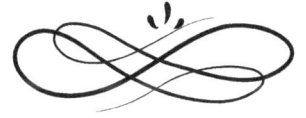

I dedicate this book to my parents, Chris and Jean Foster. Thank you for giving me this life and helping shape me into the person I am today.

Testimonials

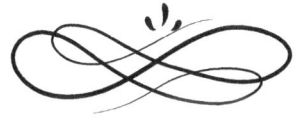

"When I first met Rachael, she really struggled to have a conversation with me and I would have to repeat myself over and over again because she would drift off or not comprehend what I was saying. Rach was also physically, mentally and emotionally weak with poor boundaries, believing she was going to be stuck for the rest of her life in a broken state.

In the short time I have known Rach, I have watched her go from a broken-down woman into a woman with strength, courage, intelligence, and professionalism. She's become an inspiration and role model to all those who believe they are stuck in life or will be disabled mentally, emotionally and physically.

I have so much trust and belief in Rachael after having the honour of watching her journey to become the powerhouse that she is now."

– **Chantel Mary**

"I have known Rachael for most of my life in WA. A little close to 15 years and I have never met a more down-to-earth person in my life. Rachie has been through hell and come back out on the other side still as lovely and caring as she's been throughout the whole time I have known her.

She has helped me through the toughest times I've been through and provided amazing positive feedback and stuck by my side through it all. I am so proud of how far Rachie has come."

– **Cameron Johnson**

"Our lives changed dramatically when our daughter Rachael was a passenger in a car accident. The recovery period was incredible, not just with trauma and pain management, but anxiety, depression and self-doubt that changed her. She would call me up in the middle of a meltdown, having a panic attack and I would try to my best ability to calm her down and talk her through it.

It was hard as parents to hear medical professionals doubting her and asking her the same questions over and over, like if she really was in pain, if this was all in her mind, or if she was seeking various medication prescriptions.

During her recovery period, Rachael discovered alternative medications and started doing courses such as hypnotherapy. Since this time, she has become much calmer, relaxed and can manage her outbursts. Her feelings do not get out of control and she no longer loses the ability to think clearly. She is a much happier and more positive person—more like the Rach we had before. I feel that we are blessed to still have her and love her very much."

– **Jean & Chris Foster (Mum and Dad)**

"Rachael has had a lot of ups and downs throughout her life. The car accident she had in 2018 was one of her biggest challenges, which tested her physically and mentally. During this time, I saw her fall deep into a struggle of pain, anxiety, depression, and a lack of hope. I watched her try various medications, which never seemed to make much difference to her mental health and how she was feeling.

When Rachael started to explore alternative therapies like hypnotherapy, I noticed a shift in her thought patterns and energy toward life. Before alternative therapies, Rachael struggled to control her emotions, often leading to outbursts that she would later regret. At times, she was crippled by her anxiety and frustration with life, which left her feeling unmotivated and unhappy.

Her growth over the past years since receiving and practicing alternative therapies has been exponential. Rachael no longer lets her emotions fuel her. She instead channels a calming and positive energy within herself to control how she is feeling. She has shifted her way of thinking and her outlook on life. This has had a positive impact on the relationships in her life and how she handles the challenges she faces. She has become resilient, strong, and most importantly, happy."

– **Liz**

"I have known Rach for many years now and know about the fact that she survived a near-fatal car crash and made a full recovery both mentally and physically, but this moment for me really shows how far Rach has come in the last few years. I went to visit her in hospital following a surgery she had for a broken arm. Whilst there visiting, a nurse came into the room and looked at Rach and said, 'I looked after you when you were in intensive care following that car accident you were in. You are very lucky to be alive after the injuries you sustained and to see you now and see how you have recovered is absolutely amazing.'"

– **Alessandra Burgum**

Contents

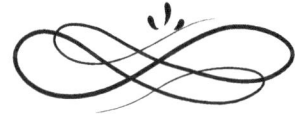

Dedication	iii
Testimonials	v
Introduction	1
Chapter One: Backstory	5
Chapter Two: Recovery	17
Chapter Three: Hypnotised	29
Chapter Four: Setback	35
Chapter Five: Dragon Magic	47
Chapter Six: Reiki Hands	63
Chapter Seven: Reiki Master	77
Chapter Eight: Colour Mirrors	85
Chapter Nine: Crystals and Metaphysics	101
Chapter Ten: Go Within	115
Chapter Eleven: Physical Vessel	127
Chapter Twelve: No Mistakes	143
Afterword	157
About the Author	159
References	163
Further Testimonials	165

Introduction

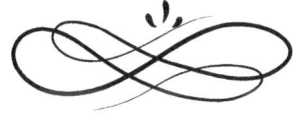

I have written this book with the intention to help people who have experienced trauma or difficulties in their life. Ideally, people who are open-minded and want to help themselves. Those who are ready to transform themselves and their lives.

I wrote this book to inspire and help others so that they can feel inspired to turn their life around. I also want this book to teach more people about alternate therapies that aren't in the mainstream. I believe these therapies are valuable and can help many people, as they did me. I hope that this book provides a different perspective on healing and life itself. One that may not be as widely understood yet.

As the reader, feel free to use this book to gain insight into energetic healing, and to feel inspired that you can overcome life's challenges. I hope that this book can guide you toward the desired change in your life, or at least give you hope that it's possible for you to transform your life. It's never too late to rewrite your story from a traumatic past into a triumphant present and future.

The overall message I want to convey is that you're not necessarily stuck just because mainstream therapies or healthcare say so. There's a whole hidden world out there waiting to be explored!

I delayed my time writing this book as at one stage, I convinced myself that I'm better off hiding away and remaining private. I have since realised that my story and perspective are valuable today and need to be shared now. In 2022, the year I'm writing, current health systems, including mental health, are experiencing high demand. Society seems to be getting more stressed and sicker as the world around us forges ahead with "business as usual". The time we have is now, why hold back?

As somebody who used to despise life and felt trapped bouncing around therapy programs and practitioners, I have truly become humbled by the very thing I once hated: life. After taking responsibility for my well-being, I'm now so appreciative of everything I have experienced and overcome. I'm grateful for the person I've become today. Out of this gratitude, I want to share some of my stories and insights to reveal that solutions are possible. Things really can improve (as cliché as it sounds). I used to roll my eyes at that statement.

I would also like to say thank you for opening this book and giving me the chance to share my story and learnings with you. I don't want to come across as I think I'm right and everything else is wrong. This is just my perspective of the world and what I have experienced.

I hope in some way this book inspires you to at least be open to there being alternative perspectives in life. There's more than one way of viewing or understanding something. We all experience life differently.

Introduction

You may find yourself presented with some foreign ideas, such as my belief that we're so much more than our physical bodies. I also believe that everything around us is bursting with life. Everything is so interconnected, including our Earth and the galaxies.

You just have to breathe the air in to feel it. How alive we and everything around us really is. Alive with pure, divine love energy.

I could be called a fool, and I do accept that. I'm not aiming to be a guru or right in my views. I'm simply telling my story, not claiming to know more than anyone else.

Everyone has a different view and experience in life.

Here's mine.

Thank you for taking the time to read about it.

Chapter One

Backstory

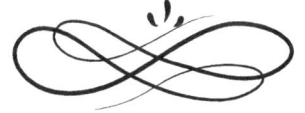

"Life is a journey and not a destination."
– Ralph Waldo Emerson, Aerosmith

I'm sure we all have very fond memories of being a child and the carefree lifestyle. Life was simple for most. My life was pretty simple back then. I had my fair share of challenges, which I'm sure we all do whilst growing up. Still, every person is born with a dualistic nature for we live in a dualistic universe. This means there are both positive and negative energies. There are dark and light energies, I should say. Whether something is positive or negative, it still helps us grow. Also, there's a negative in every positive, like there's a positive in every negative. It's all about perspective. We need one in order to have the other, otherwise, none would exist.

So even if you had a perfect childhood, there still would have been instances that you viewed as wrong or bad and that would have created what we call a childhood wound. You would have internalized this, so it impacted your choices and behaviour throughout your life. I know that my parents did the best that they could for me to the best of their abilities.

I will admit that for years, I held a lot of anger and resentment towards them because I believed that certain things should and shouldn't have happened. I'm grateful that I have now made peace with these things.

I can recognize that they've made me who I am today. I know it sounds cliché, but they really did. I have reached a level of self-acceptance and self-love, so I wouldn't have my upbringing any other way. I'm proud of the person they raised me to be. I was quite a gifted and sensitive child. My parents invested a lot of time and energy into my younger years to help me be academically smart.

I was definitely that child who was a high achiever, ambitious and dedicated to my work. Although I was a high achiever, I was quite shy. But my dad also did drill into me from a young age to always stay humble, no matter what I achieve.

When I finished primary school, I went to high school not too far from where I'd grown up. I spent my first year in high school there and I continued to get good grades. I wasn't the popular kid. I had a couple of friends and me being the introvert that I was, I was happy with quality, not quantity.

By the time I reached ninth grade, I was 14 and the teenage hormones had well and truly kicked in. My parents had decided to send me to a Catholic all-girls school about an hour and a half commute from where I lived.

Up in the city. The big smoke. It was all so alien and foreign to a young girl who had spent her entire life in Rockingham and Mandurah. I remember I was driven to this fancy school to go and sit an exam to be awarded an academic scholarship. I felt sick inside. I was not excited about this at all. It wasn't exam anxiety. I was quite confident in academics. I had just gone through a bit of a shock leaving my small primary school and entering a big high school with hardly anyone I knew attending. I felt like I had just overcome this challenge by eventually making friends. I was happy with where I was. To have to start that all over again, in a city which I was not familiar with, was so scary at the time for a shy, nervous girl like me.

Amongst that, an all-girls school made me very anxious as growing up, I was quite a tomboy. I tended to have more male friends than female. I loved playing sports and I was kind of one of the boys.

I remember I sat down in this exam room and there were five girls, including myself. Three scholarships were being awarded. I felt nervous sitting in this fancy, formal classroom. It felt extra-terrestrial compared to the laidback schooling I'd grown up in. I remember thinking *I'm just going to purposely answer a fair few of these questions wrong.* I didn't want to win a scholarship. I remember skipping out of that exam room thinking, *you beauty, you got this. Nailed it. Definitely not going to pass that.*

Then, lo and behold, hello.

I don't remember how long it was until we got the feedback, but I had won the scholarship.

I remember begging my mum to not let me go. My parents said it would be a really great opportunity and that I'm so intelligent. I needed to be challenged more as I had, "So much future potential."

I will never forget my dad saying, "If you can survive an elite Catholic all-girls school, you can survive anything in life."

In hindsight, he was correct. I have proven to myself I can survive anything. I'm not sure how much the all-girls Catholic school actually contributed to that survival though.

So at the age of 14, I started at this school where you wear the little hats like in the French 90s cartoon, *Madeline*. Pretty much that, except the girls were wealthy rather than orphans. We even had nuns at our school!

Looking back, I can say obviously I was supposed to attend that school. Yet throughout my time there, I felt like an alien. I didn't quite get along with these girls. I won't go into too much detail about my schooling years. You can probably imagine what a school filled with teenage levels of estrogen and next to no testosterone would have been like. Ladies, we may say that a world with only women would be perfect. Trust me, it wouldn't. Believe it or not, we need men to balance things out.

I met my first serious boyfriend at 14. We dated for about two years. It wasn't all bad, but it was quite a controlling and socially isolating experience. He was a jealous guy. He would tell me what I could and couldn't wear. He didn't let me have male friends (he actually deleted all my mate's numbers out of my phone one day). I didn't have social media so I lost contact with a lot of them. I already didn't have many friends at my new school either.

By 16, I felt isolated and lonely. In the end, he cheated on me with another girl. He was actually trying to date her but wasn't leaving me either. How ironic.

I do appreciate the overall experience though. He was my first love and I will forever cherish the moments we had together. I definitely learnt a lot too. My key lesson from all of it was to never let a man control or dictate what's best for me. I also learnt that there's no point in being jealous or in doing things to prevent a man from cheating on you. If he's going to cheat, it doesn't matter what you do, he will cheat. It has more to do with his character than anything to do with you as a person. Of course, it still crushed me inside for years.

When I was 16 and still dating said boyfriend, I also went through a sexual assault. I had frozen in panic during the ordeal. I felt violated, dirty and ashamed for a long time. This eventually led to me learning to embrace my sexuality. I learned that a sexual assault doesn't make me unworthy, nor do I need to be ashamed. I also learnt to love my own body, despite it being mishandled in the past. This experience also taught me about gut feelings and not being afraid to leave or say no if I'm uncomfortable.

Throughout my teenage years, I did come to realise I had significant mental health issues. There were several reasons for this, some of which I've mentioned already. I had quite low self-esteem. I was depressed and self-harming. I felt helpless and wanted to die. I think the only thing that really kept me going was the hope that life would get better after high school. I'm sure a lot of us hoped that. Teenage years can be brutal, even for the best of us.

By year 12, I was 17 and diagnosed with anxiety. That was something I'd apparently had since being a young child. It seemed so normal to me. I didn't even realise that not everyone was extremely stressed like I was.

Back then, mental health was not as widely understood as it is today. My parents didn't understand it or know how to help. Like most of my generation's parents, it was such a foreign concept. I ended up feeling ashamed and like there was something wrong with me. I didn't understand why I couldn't just be like the other kids. Why did every day feel like a battle with my mind?

I did well at masking it all. I poured myself into school work, painting, playing guitar and video games in order to distract myself from the mental mess I existed in. I went on to battle with severe mental health issues for about a decade.

What I mostly learnt from all of it was that it's okay to admit you're struggling. That it's okay to admit I'm not perfect. The more I talked about it, the more I connected with other people. This helped me realise I wasn't alone. I wasn't some freak or alien that battles with themselves frequently. It's actually quite normal and most of us do experience at least some sort of phase of poor mental health during our lifetime.

After graduating high school, I attended university and started a four-year psychology degree. I was accepted into a graduate with honours pool based on my final results. All I had to do was maintain a GPA of 3.0 out of 4.0 throughout the degree, which I did. Even alongside partying and late nights working at a night club as a bartender.

Halfway through my third year of the degree, I shocked my family and friends by deciding to change my degree to a Bachelor of Arts in Psychology. In order to become a registered psychologist,

I would need to also complete my Master's in Psychology. I was on track to get into a Master's program being an honours student. Nobody understood why.

So what changed in my third year? I had discovered psychedelics.

LSD and psilocybin opened my mind to a lot of realisations. It led to me having a spiritual awakening. One realisation was that I had spent my whole life doing what I was told to do or what was expected of me. Not once had I asked myself what I was actually passionate about in life.

I received the award for the top grades in psychology in year 12. I had no idea what I actually wanted to do when I left school except that I wanted to help people somehow. I decided to study to be a psychologist based on this simple fact. I had always lived my life for my parents, trying to make them proud and happy. I had made a lot of life decisions based on what I believed they wanted.

I could no longer understand why I was doing a degree when it wasn't my passion in life. I had this vision of myself being miserable in this job, but then feeling obliged to keep working in it because of the good salary to pay off the debt, that I'd put myself in for the degree.

At the time it all sounded like madness to those on the outside. Heck, I even questioned if it was madness or if I was onto something here. I felt this inner conviction that I had a different calling in life. I didn't know what it was, but I knew what it was not.

Despite fumbling around for years not knowing what direction I was headed, I'm so glad I trusted my gut instinct in my early 20s. It's gotten me to this exact moment. I can truly say, at the age of 27, I'm doing what I love and I genuinely enjoy what I do.

My advice to any teenager leaving school would be, don't do a job because society expects you to, or because it looks good on paper. Find and follow what you're passionate about.

My advice to any adult feeling stuck in a job they despise is to work towards another pathway. Follow your passions and dreams, life is too short to not live on the terms you want to. Where there's a will, there's a way. Don't give up on your dreams.

So, I early exit graduated from university at the age of 20 with a Bachelor of Arts in Psychology. Around this time, I also met a guy who was seven years older than me. I had boyfriends before, but this one absolutely swept me off my feet. I had never felt so adored and special to a man before. Every day felt like a wonderful adventure with him. I finally felt accepted and understood. There were some major red flags, though I had pushed them to the side as I was blinded by love.

After about three months, his patience started wearing thin. He would snap at me or explode in a rage yelling. It used to frighten me a lot. I would bring it up and his response would be to minimise things by saying, "Well at least I didn't hit you, that's what a real abusive boyfriend would do." I would accept that and ignore my own inner voice.

As time went on, he did start getting violent with me. Eventually, it got as bad as strangling me until I blacked out. I ended up with PTSD from nearly dying at the hands of a lover. Despite my attempts to leave, I would go back. My self-esteem had been ruined and I felt so dependent on him. It was like he was the only person I felt safe with, but ironically, he was the one causing the most harm.

I couldn't see it though. Maybe it was some form of Stockholm Syndrome, or maybe I genuinely believed he was going to change.

Backstory

I didn't want to give up on this man. I would see flickers of the generous, caring man I'd fallen in love with. It would give me hope that he was making progress with his own inner demons.

During this time, I had several different jobs. Due to my poor mental health from being abused, I couldn't hold any down. I was very loyal to this man and wanted to support him despite sacrificing my own well-being in the process. I can see how we both were toxic to each other in some ways. I'm not going to sit here and say I was a victim and play the blame game. I take responsibility for my part in staying and turning a blind eye. This man did hide his methamphetamine use from me, which, at the time people did say it was obvious but I just wanted to see the good. I had ignored what my gut was telling me.

This relationship went on for nearly a year. I'll never forget my dad crying on Christmas Day, asking me to please get rid of this guy because I deserve so much better. I knew he was right. I had put him before my own needs and well-being. I didn't want to abandon him when I could see he was in a really dark place. I was too self-sacrificing in a way. However, it all sunk in seeing how much it was emotionally affecting my dad. I will never forget hearing him say how he wanted me to date a guy who he can be best friends with and take fishing. Someone he can do dude stuff with because he never had any sons.

Dad said he can't be best friends with this guy. I understood that as this guy couldn't even be friends with my own friends, let alone my father. I went home after Christmas to see this guy like me and him had agreed upon earlier. As usual, he started going off about something. I grabbed my bag and I just ran out the door with him chasing me. I jumped in my car and drove away. I had finally found the strength to leave.

Despite blocking his number, he repeatedly called to threaten and beg for me from a No Caller ID number. I will admit I did eventually go spend time with him again as I was quite co-dependent and he would promise that he had changed. It would turn to shit every time though.

In the end, I wanted to be left alone and was granted a Violence Restraining Order (VRO). But in his words, a piece of paper wasn't going to keep him away from the woman he loves. The calls would continue. The police counted 300 in the space of one hour. This went on for two weeks until the police finally arrested him for breaching the VRO.

I was relieved when he was arrested. I was terrified for my life. Not because I thought this guy was a murderer, but because I knew he was really unwell. He was heavy on the drugs and couldn't let me go. I was concerned he would accidentally commit a passion crime due to feeling so intense about me leaving him.

He had already strangled me until I passed out. I thought that I had died. I went limp. He had already done that a few months prior to me trying to break up with him. I was terrified.

I don't regret that experience. It taught me about having healthy boundaries and not living in co-dependency. It also taught me to not make excuses for someone's poor behaviour. I won't ever fall in love with future potential, now I focus on the present. I learnt my worth, and also about tough love. I also learnt to put myself first.

After he went to jail, I had a psychotic breakdown. The doctors said it was because I had gone into autopilot survival mode whilst he was abusing me. My brain wasn't processing my emotions fully so it could protect me from the extremes I had been living with. I was dissociating so that I wouldn't have a mental breakdown and be in possibly more danger. The moment he was locked up, I was safe to break down.

I was put on medications to cope. By this point, my spirituality had gotten to a point where I was connecting with the unseen world and picking up on messages from this realm. I could feel the spirit world supporting me and celebrating me despite this trauma. I would cycle through feeling scared and down to feeling euphoric and on top of the world.

Doctors said I was having a manic episode triggered by stress and also a bad reaction to the medications. I was then prescribed anti-psychotics and returned to my friend's house. I had been staying there as I didn't feel safe at my place. There I ended up regressing into a younger version of myself and apparently, it was like I was two or three. At this point, my friend's mother said I needed to go to the hospital and be an inpatient. I went along with it and ended up in a mental ward. I'm not saying that psych wards are bad, but it didn't work for me.

I didn't seem to be improving. I was becoming more of a shell and I was shutting down. Due to the antipsychotic medications, I couldn't feel my connection with the spirit world anymore. I felt completely alone. The way patients were treated in the ward was quite dehumanising. One lady I had befriended in there comforted me one day after I had a breakdown.

I'll never forget what she told me: "Rachael, you're not sick. There's nothing wrong with you. It's society. Society is sick."

At that point, I realised I needed to return to my normal life as being at the ward seemed to be sending me backwards. Luckily, I was a voluntary patient so I minimised my symptoms and said I was okay. I went home within about four or five days and resumed my work at the nightclub when I felt ready to.

Around this time I set up my art business *Art by iluka* as I found painting to really help me with the trauma. I found out I had complex PTSD. Originally, I thought I had borderline personality disorder, which was diagnosed whilst I was being abused. Later on, a psychologist said no way do I have that or I wouldn't be able to function with living alone for the two years I had at the time. I didn't have a fear of abandonment either.

My dad took me on a holiday to Thailand and Vietnam, as he suggested it would help me more than psych wards and medications. That trip really did set my soul free, and it awakened a travel bug within me.

Six months after, I got a new job at a pub. My goal was to save enough money and travel the world. I wanted to explore. I still had no idea what I wanted to do for a career. Plus, now I had all this extra trauma to live with. I was a nervous wreck, and I wanted to find myself again through travel.

However, that didn't go to plan. Another six months later, I was the passenger in a major car accident. I hit my head badly and had to learn how to walk again.

But, despite it all, this story actually has a happy ending.

Chapter Two

Recovery

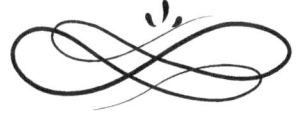

"The more I draw and write, the more I realise that accidents are a necessary part of any creative act, much more so than logic or wisdom. Sometimes a mistake is the only way of arriving at an original concept, and the history of successful inventions is full of mishaps, serendipity and unintended results."

– Shaun Tan

It was all very surreal waking up in the hospital after the crash. I was groggy and confused. It all felt like a really bad nightmare. Eventually, the reality of it all kicked in. I was in the ICU on a drip being fed Fentanyl. I looked down and was relieved to see my leg was still there. I had been told it may have needed to be amputated due to the complicated breaks in my femur and hip joint.

You learn how to walk as a kid. Well, most children do. It's something you never think about because it's so automatic and part of the process of growing up and developing.

I never pictured that I would have to learn how to walk again. As an adult, I definitely took my legs for granted. I took my ability to walk for granted. Which is fair enough. Most of us don't think about it, do we? It wasn't until something so simple, yet so necessary, was taken from me that I realized how ungrateful I had been about the important things.

How bitter, angry and upset I had been about things that actually didn't really matter that much in the grand scheme of things. I think one of my favourite sayings nowadays is, "If it's not something you're going to worry about in five years, or even one year's time, it's not even worth worrying about."

This is coming from me, who used to absolutely lose my shit if the smallest thing in my home was out of place.

Being trapped in the car was very horrific. I don't remember much of the actual crash. I couldn't really see as there was blood pouring down my face from hitting my head. All I could smell was blood. I found it difficult to breathe as thick, red sludge was entering my nose. I didn't even notice my leg at first. I was in shock.

Prior to the accident, I remember looking down at my phone. Then, everything was black. As if I was asleep.

Then it was like I woke up. I was disorientated because I'd realised the car had stopped. I had this splitting headache.

I was confused and panicked. I put my hand to my forehead. I noticed my eyebrow was dangling and wet. I realised I was bleeding.

Recovery

As soon as I tried to get out of the car, my leg was in agony. I couldn't move. I'd never broken a bone up until this point. I had no idea what was happening. The pain was kicking in intensely. It was the worst pain I had experienced in my life. From what I heard, I was quite angry and screaming. I hardly remember that.

The time being stuck in that car felt like a lifetime. Waiting for the fire brigade to come and cut me out of the vehicle with no pain relief felt like an eternity.

I'm so grateful that none of us died. I don't know where I would be today if a life had been lost that night. As tragic as it was, I still think it could have been so much worse. I do believe that night there was a guardian angel. It's a miracle that I wasn't amputated from the hip or that I didn't lose my eye as the scarring goes down into my eye socket.

Being in the hospital is also blurry for me because I'd hit my head quite badly. I was also on a lot of painkillers. I'm so grateful for nurses and doctors and medical teams. They're amazing people.

I spent a month in rehab learning how to walk again. I was really ambitious at the time. My outlook was quite positive. At the time of the accident, I was off psych meds and had been reconnecting with the spirit realms. I had already done a bit of self-development at this point. I knew mind over matter and I wanted to not let this break me. I believed in myself.

I could see though, that everyone around me was shocked. They were broken to see me this way. I could see the pain in everyone who looked at me. Some people couldn't even really look at me or visit me. I understand. It's a hard reality. It's confronting. It was confronting for me as well. I took it on board. I didn't want to worry anybody. I didn't want to make a fuss. I made sure to try and keep strong for everyone around me, not just myself.

I had screws inserted into my hip, a rod inserted along my femur and more screws inserted into my kneecap to hold the bones together. I was told there was a chance that the blood supply in my hip would be cut off and I may need a hip replacement in a few years time.

It took me around four months to actually come off crutches and begin walking. As I was a bartender at the time, I started a new job in a law firm. However, we didn't realise that my concussion was more than a concussion.

I actually had slowed processing in my brain. I really struggled at this job. At the same time, I had doctors telling me that it wasn't a mild brain injury and that I was perfectly fine. Well, yes, I did appear on the outside to be perfectly fine. There was no structurally significant brain damage. However, it's not unheard of for cognitive issues to occur from a major impact to the head and there not be any structural damage.

I knew that my brain didn't work like this before the accident. I knew myself better than anybody or any doctor. Yes, I had smoked cannabis in my life and maybe had some party drugs. But it wasn't like this before the accident or after being strangled by my ex. I could still function very well with my organisational skills.

I knew myself. Something had changed.

It was like I couldn't access the vocabulary that I used to. I'd forgotten big words. It was like anything more than one or two, maybe three syllables, I had forgotten. I was not as literate as I used to be.

I knew something was wrong. No way would I have been able to finish my university degree with the grades I had if this is how my brain always was. I was highly intelligent. This was not me. And the doctors just compared me to the average of everybody else and said, "Well you can tick these boxes. You're fine."

Yes, but something was wrong. My abilities had deteriorated. This is not how I used to be. But as far as they were concerned, I was functional and it didn't matter. I could still hold down a job. I wasn't brain-dead.

That devastated me. It was like it didn't even matter, yet it really mattered to me. I felt like not only had my physical body been taken, but so had my mental capacity. I felt like a number in the system. A statistic, not a person.

Once I was given the all-clear medically with my hip, I returned back to bar work. At first, it worked out, but over time, the limp I had worsened. The pain was increasing.

I remember telling my doctor. I was told that it shouldn't be like that and it was in my head. That it was a psychological pain because the X-rays weren't coming back with anything. My doctor wasn't interested in doing any further investigations.

What I struggled with the most with the medical system was that all of my issues were looked at separately by different doctors. I wasn't an entire person.

I was my muscular system to my physio. I was my bones to my surgeon. I was my mental health to my psychologist and later psychiatrist. I was never Rach. I was never the soul living in my physical body that was experiencing thoughts and emotions. I was never looked at as a whole entity. I was segmented and separated into damaged pieces of my former self.

My main discovery from this experience is how important it is to step back and look at the bigger picture when it comes to health and well-being. It's necessary to integrate everything holistically. Different aspects interrelate and influence each other. People aren't just their "leg" or "depression".

As my limp got worse, and the pain worsened, so did my mental health. I got increasingly stressed. Nobody really believed me about my cognitive issues, except close loved ones. This caused more stress, which then made my cognitive issues worse, which then also made the physical pain worse.

It was this vicious cycle that I had no awareness of at the time. I just thought there was something wrong with me. These doctors were the experts. I was looking to them and believing they could help me. I needed them to help me, I was in the worst pain of my life. I can't even describe it. It was pure hell. I just wanted it to stop.

I was taking so many painkillers to the point where my doctor one day said that I was abusing them. He thought I had a painkiller addiction and said if I didn't slow down, he was going to stop prescribing them. At this stage, I had already been cut back to only Panadeine forte. It was not doing much for me. I was prescribed to take eight a day. I was taking eight every two hours and I was still in pain.

I was so dysfunctional because of it. I was bedridden. But I was so determined. I didn't want to give up. I still went to work even though bartending had become a struggle. I was told to keep up or I wasn't trying because I couldn't recall the new menu. I was honestly forgetful.

Recovery

I remember I would walk out and sit in the toilets. I would have to sit there and just rest. I would hide in there to rest my hip. I would breathe and cry. I would try to pull it together. Since I was young, I could never cry in front of people. I found it weak to do that.

I believed this was all my mental health. The pain was not really there physically. *How fucked up is my brain?* I used to think, as I would recall all my lifelong battles of being at war with my mind.

I struggled to even tell people how I was really doing except for those who were closest to me. I felt so weak. I felt like a failure. I didn't give up. I didn't want to give myself a break. But I think I was slowly giving up.

Because of the agony I was in, I was taking so many painkillers so I could work. The side effects from the meds were also making me too sick to work the hours I was. However, I really needed the money to survive as well.

I was so determined to return to normal, yet almost in denial. I was listening to my doctors and they were telling me that I had to work. Three months after the accident, my doctor wouldn't let me be on the medical pension with Centrelink. He said I was fit to work. Despite the extreme amount of pain I was living with, I believed him.

Eventually, my shifts were cut down to about one or two a week. I understand because I was not fit to be working in that environment. They needed more reliable people during their busiest time of the year.

Not being on any government allowance, I was now desperate for income.

I saw an ad on Facebook for a job as a skimpy barmaid for double my hourly rate. Working as a contractor under an ABN, being my own boss, and choosing my own hours with short shifts. I decided to give it a go. Never in my life did I think I would work in the adult industry.

I kept it very hidden for a long time, especially from family, because of the stigma. I felt ashamed to be in that line of work. I'm not anymore. I'm proud. People can think what they want. There's nothing wrong with that kind of work. It's actually very empowering and liberating for a woman. Any feminist that tries to say that it's not is actually being sexist and denying women's freedom.

If men want to give us good money for that, and we're following our own boundaries, just because they're different from maybe another woman's boundaries, it doesn't mean there's anything wrong with it. Yes, I worked in my underwear and naked but nobody was allowed to touch me in personal areas because of my boundaries. Some women are different and that's okay too. I personally couldn't, but I still got judged and called horrible names to my face and behind my back by people that I thought were my friends.

At the end of the day, I gained so much confidence despite my injuries. The men were really supportive and understanding. They had a lot of respect for me to be walking around with this limp and extreme pain from a major car accident. To not be giving up. To not be sitting around on the dole. To still be out there giving it a fair go and doing the best I could with the cards that I had been dealt.

Yes, every now and then you get an asshole. Though I was actually pretty surprised the majority of the guys were respectful and understanding of me. Quite often I found working in those bars, a lot of them just want someone to listen or someone to connect with.

It's not about sex. Yes, you're a pretty girl and they're attracted to you. But it's the connection that they appreciate. It's the fun and the laughter and the entertainment that you provide.

I had a lot of fun. It helped lift my spirits. I was also paid to travel and see more of Western Australia than I had ever seen in my whole life. However, as this went on, the pain was getting more excruciating. I was getting frantic.

By then, I was starting to get aggressive, angry and really snapping at people in my life. I had no patience. I was in so much pain. It took all my strength to be living in that pain. The littlest thing was going to send me over. Plus, I still had this unresolved PTSD from the previous abusive relationship. My partner at the time was my rock and I treated him, my mother and my father probably the worst.

Isn't that ironic? How we treat the people closest to us the worst sometimes. I do appreciate them sticking by me and seeing past it. I do feel remorseful for my attitude and the things I said and did out of rage and frustration. It wasn't their fault, but I tried to make it their fault and problem. My relationships did break down; it all took a toll.

The physical and mental pain became so unbearable one night, I drank alcohol and swallowed a heap of pills to try to OD. It didn't work. I think that's what annoyed me the most. Waking back up and going, *Fuck I'm still here. I'm that useless, I can't even kill myself correctly.*

As time went on, my leg went from one centimetre to two centimetres shorter. The pain was worsening as time continued. I was still being told the pain was neurological by my doctor. My surgeon was saying it was probably the metal in my hip so I was on a waitlist to get it removed. I was told by my physio that sometimes when you break a bone, you lose a bit of it and unfortunately, that's what's happened to me. I needed a fitting in my shoe. I'll just have uneven legs for the rest of my life.

It devastated me. I thought I was permanently stuck with a limp. Eventually, I got to that breaking point and I snapped. I remember I wrote a note to my family, saying I'm sorry. I love them. Please don't blame yourself. I'm at peace now. Because I can't live in this pain anymore. I got drunk and I drove my car off the road in an attempt to finish the job that I believed the first accident should have done.

I just couldn't understand why the fuck I hadn't died in the first crash. What kind of sick twisted joke it was that I was still alive. Why would the universe keep me here? Surviving. Barely. Just let me rest and be at peace.

I remember crashing the car into the bushes off the road and swearing because I, again, failed. It didn't come close to anything like the first accident. I did write my car off. I was arrested and charged with drunk driving. I lost my license and now had to walk even more.

The police didn't really believe that I was suicidal. I was taken to the hospital for assessment. I was in a terrible place mentally. I was so over struggling and feeling as if the whole world was against me.

Eventually, I was discharged and I went back to my partner at the time's home and passed out. I woke up in the morning and felt so horrible. The reality of my actions the night before was really kicking in.

In hindsight, I understand I wasn't supposed to die back then. I had a bigger purpose. The spirit world wasn't going to let this end here. Everything happens for a reason. I'm a true believer in that. I can now use all of these experiences to help others going through something similar. Sharing hardships is one way we can relate and connect with each other.

In less than a week, I had this appointment with a new surgeon because I had decided to get a second opinion upon my aunty's recommendation. She found a good surgeon who specialised in orthopaedics for young people. I did have a mental breakdown the day before going to the appointment. I had given up. I couldn't even walk to the doctor. I collapsed outside the front of the hospital with my mother. I was put in a wheelchair and taken up by Mum as she was saying, "Come on, we got this, let's do this."

I was saying, "There's no point, they're just going to tell me that there's nothing wrong. I'm stuck like this."

To my surprise, the surgeon took me seriously and listened to me. He sent me for a CT scan of my hip. When those results came back in, we sat down and I'll never forget how validating that moment was for me.

He said, "Rachael, your pain is very real. You're in an incredible amount of pain. We are going to fix this. It's fixable."

I found out that I had necrosis in my hip, and my hip joint had completely died. The top of my femur had also died. This was from a lack of blood supply. Within five days I had hip replacement surgery. I was 24.

After my hip replacement, I made a full recovery. I was able to walk. I still had tenderness and pain. However, I think after the whole ordeal, the pain had become psychological because it lingered on further than it should have. I was still taking lots of painkillers.

Eventually, I had a neurologist take me seriously and recommend me for some cognitive therapy and I did a bit of brain rehab for about a year. I improved, but I still wasn't 100%. Same as the pain I was in. I still wasn't 100%. Though, it was a lot better than what it had been.

I definitely have learnt to trust my own instincts about my body and mind. Always get a second or third opinion if doctors aren't listening.

Chapter Three

Hypnotised

"You have the power to heal your life, and you need to know that. We think so often that we are helpless, but we're not. We always have the power of our minds… claim and consciously use your power."

– Louise L. Hay

It's interesting how the people we meet can send us on a whole new trajectory in life. How one small action can completely change the course of our lives.

Whilst I had been away working in Kalgoorlie, I had come across a crystal store. I saw these adorable crystal wolf pendants and posted them on my Instagram story. One was tiger eye, which I bought for myself. The other type was amethyst.

One lady, Chantel, whom I knew through the adult entertainment industry replied to my story asking if I could buy her the amethyst wolf pendant. She sent me the money to buy it straight away. I remember thinking, *whoa that is a lot of trust. How does she know I won't just run off with the cash?* We had never actually met personally.

I bought it for her. When I got back to Perth, she came to my house to pick it up and we met in person. Outside the front of my place, we had a chat. She asked me what my goals were in the industry and what I was planning to do with my future. Obviously, we were on good money, yet I had no goal other than to survive and have fun at that point.

Realistically, if you want to be smart in this industry, you use your income to invest in something else, like a small business or to pay for school. Me, I was just working this job to survive and pay my bills. I wasn't even really working that many hours. I felt embarrassed to admit my current health condition, so I responded by saying I hadn't really thought about it.

Chantel's response was something along the lines of, "Well, this isn't a very good environment for anyone long term, but also you practice spirituality. All of the dark, toxic energies they're going to be wanting to attach to your light and happy people don't sit around in pubs drinking so you'll be absorbing those energies. You need a plan. Use this money to build something so you can move forward in life."

At the time, I didn't quite comprehend what she meant. But I did sort of understand. At this point, the job was draining me physically, mentally and emotionally.

One day, Chantel messaged me offering a free ticket for a hypnotherapy course. I jumped on board, as I thought, *why not? This could be a good opportunity. I've already got a Bachelor of Arts in Psychology. It's a free ticket. It's not like if I'm too stupid to learn this it will really matter.*

I showed up to the event. I was really anxious and nervous. My confidence had been shot and this was the first educational classroom-type activity I had done in a long time. In this course, I learnt about the power of the mind and beliefs.

I learnt how beliefs can impact our minds, and influence our feelings and behaviour. I also learnt that these beliefs can be "reprogrammed" and that we aren't just "stuck" a certain way. We're not slaves to our thoughts, in fact, we aren't even our thoughts at all. We're the observer of our thoughts.

Over that weekend, we got to pick something we wanted to shift during the course. Mine was to quit smoking cigarettes. It was successful. I'd wanted to quit smoking cigarettes. I had tried. You know the age-old story. I just couldn't seem to shake it. The hypnotherapy did help me quit smoking for 18 months. I'll be honest, I did relapse when I was drunk. It unravelled my progress because apparently, that's the thing with quitting smoking from hypnosis. From all of this, I have learnt that hypnosis is powerful, however, we still actively make our decisions as well, so don't think being hypnotised once will delete old patterns permanently.

As Chantel later explained to me, you need to understand why you're doing the behaviour in the first place, otherwise, the work you did removing and replacing belief systems can unravel. Conscious awareness of the why is important.

At the end of the course, after we got our certificates, I got talking to Chantel more. I opened up about the car accident, about how I had slowed cognitive abilities and was still in pain even though the pain had also improved after the hip replacement. I was still experiencing pain, fatigue, anxiety and depression. I didn't even mention the DV and PTSD at this point.

She suggested I book in with her for a session as she could use kinesiology and hypnotherapy on me to help. At this point, I was keen to try anything. I had already tried to do everything through the medical system and still felt broken.

I was so nervous and scared going to see her at the beginning. I didn't know what to expect. I could tell this lady was really spiritual. At that point, I had a lot of shame about my past and fear of judgment. I was a bit scared she would be able to read my mind or be able to just see everything inside of my brain and know everything about me. I wouldn't be able to hide it all. That did scare me but I was so desperate to try anything that could possibly help me.

Chantel was confident that we would be able to work through this and that the body can heal itself. That the power of the mind is unlimited. What you believe is what will come true. But simply just telling yourself to believe didn't quite help in my experience. Well, it could, but it's a longer process. You need to get to the blueprint of your mind, the subconscious mind. Shifts at a subconscious level help speed up the process of change. Otherwise, you're only looking at a small little piece of the puzzle. The belief or thought.

However, everything fits together and interacts in some shape or form. We are complex beings, not just a single component that needs to be zeroed in on and that little issue gets fixed or looked at. Quite often, things are all interlinked and interrelated. They feed into each other and you need to unravel them. Not just focus on one thing.

I remember after a few sessions, I was experiencing the least amount of pain, stress and mental symptoms that I had felt in years. I was blown away. I was still a bit scared because I was worried thinking, *did she see everything that I've ever done in my life? Does she see that I'm a bad person?* At this point, I had been living with so much guilt and shame. I had this deep belief that I was a bad person. I don't even know where I picked it up from. It was probably some inner-child wound that I had somehow managed to take on board, like we do when we're young children.

That's the thing about energetic healing. It doesn't really matter what caused it. We don't need to go and play the blame game or pick the past apart. It's just, "Okay. This is the issue today. This is what's going on here. We're going to work on present-day issues and the why behind those." In doing that, it seems to then go back and unravel these deep patterns that we carry.

Overall, the main thing I learnt from connecting with Chantel in the beginning was that it's safe to trust other people and let them in. By this stage, I had lost trust in people; I was isolating myself and pushing people away because of how much pain I was in. I learnt that even a stranger can care and want to help. The world wasn't 100% against me or unfair, there are good people that exist.

I also learnt that just because something isn't 100% recognised by the medical world or society, it doesn't mean it's a scam or it won't work. I realised that the world of alternative therapies and wellness existed for a reason. It was beneficial and powerful.

Chapter Four

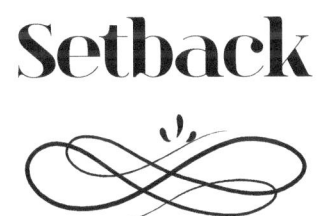

Setback

"The road to recovery is not linear. It's not straight. It's a bumpy path with lots of twists and turns. But you're on the right track."

– Candice Carty Williams

I continued to receive mostly Dragon Magic Hypnotic from Chantel. Dragon Magic Hypnotic is actually her own form of hypnotherapy that she developed. I will be discussing it in more detail in chapter five.

I was getting incredibly miraculous results after a couple of months.

You often need to have several sessions to notice much difference. It depends on how deep-rooted the issue is. It varies for everybody.

It's rarely going to be a one-session fix. We're working on, quite often, years and years of trauma, wounding, or just unhealthy habits, behaviours and thoughts. It didn't take a day for these things to happen. It's not going to take a day for them to be undone.

One of my favourite sayings is that Rome wasn't built in a day. Quite often I have had to remind myself of this, as I found myself to be quite impatient with my own healing for some time.

The pandemic happened about one month after I completed my hypnotherapy qualification. I could no longer work in the bar. We were locked down.

I remember that mentally set me back somewhat. It wasn't too bad because I'd spent a long time already in hospital. I had spent a long time bedridden, stuck at home. I thought, *well I'm stuck at home but at least this time, I'm a lot more mobile, and the whole world is with me on this—I'm not alone.*

My biggest stressor was financial. I didn't know how long it would take to return to work or whether the industry I was in would be stable again. I realised that I can't rely on a "job" or working for someone else. I needed to expand my skills and grow. I also wanted to work in something I was passionate about so that I didn't wake up dreading the day because I have work. During the pandemic, like a lot of us did, I began to re-evaluate my life. It was seeming my dreams to travel the world and find myself again were to be halted once more.

Once we were out of lockdown, I was really excited. My body was doing amazing—something I once believed impossible. I had this new 4WD and I wanted to go camping and have a holiday. So, I did with my on-and-off partner at the time.

Setback

The first night my car keys got lost. I honestly didn't know when we had lost them. I'd been drinking alcohol all afternoon and evening. Some people offered to help me look for them by driving me up the beach.

We were driving along on the sand at night in the back of the car. It was getting really bumpy and I'd had the car accident with somebody who I didn't really know driving so this experience triggered an *oh my god, I'm having an accident again* moment.

I told them to slow down and then stop and they wouldn't stop. Instead, they kind of laughed at me. They brushed it off because they didn't know I had a car accident. This is where I learned my boundaries now. I need to tell every new person I get into the car with that I've had this accident so if I do freak out this will never happen again.

What I did was thought it'd be a good idea to just open the car door and jump out. That's trauma for you. The perceived danger of having another car accident was greater than the one of jumping out of the car. I realised I was going down headfirst and thought, *oh shit, I'm gonna break my neck and end up in a wheelchair.* I somehow had time to use my left arm to brace my fall because I'm right-handed. I did not want to bust my hip again. After an ambulance trip to the hospital, I learnt I snapped my upper arm. Another very complicated break. Typical Rach at the time.

At this point, I was even traumatized by hospitals and surgery. I remember arguing and arguing with the doctors. They wanted to operate and I refused to sign the necessary forms. I made them give me a cast and sling which caused all sorts of complications over the next few months. It didn't quite heal right and I actually re-snapped half the bone six months prior to me writing this. Currently,

I have had the surgery (delays happened due to Covid). I had a metal plate and screws implanted and my arm in another sling.

So far, recovery has been really smooth. I have overcome my fear of hospitals and gained faith in my body's ability to heal. I have also let go of resentment and hatred towards the medical system. I used to think that there was no way I was going near a hospital again. However, I do understand life is about balance. We need all of it. We need spiritual energetic healing and we need medical healing too. Both serve their own purposes and both are just as important. One is not more supreme than the other.

Yes, my body could have healed my broken arm fine with another cast. However, the older I get, the more likely I am to re-break it. I don't want to be 67 years old, have a fall and snap it. The recovery process is a lot more on your body the older you get. I'm not saying it's impossible, but it's a bigger job.

I'm still having a journey of my own. Being on a healing journey doesn't mean that obstacles in life just disappear and go away. Rather, we become resilient and get better at handling them. If I had this operation when I first broke my arm, I wouldn't actually be facing this challenge whilst I'm writing this book now. Typing with one hand is slower than two.

Hindsight is an interesting thing, isn't it? We can't beat ourselves up either because we can't change the past. You can't be looking back and beating yourself up over something that can't be changed. It's the past, it's done now. We can learn from the past though in order to prevent reliving similar experiences. I accept that decision. I understand that this is all part of my journey. It's happening for a reason. I might not understand the reason today though years later, I probably will.

Setback

I remember going back to Chantel after breaking my arm. I was feeling so much shame again. I was thinking *oh my god, we've done all this work. I've come so far and now I've just gone like so far backward. What the heck is going on?* I felt like a failure. I was beating myself up so hard. I hadn't mentioned my internal dialogue yet, she just looked at me and said, "So what are you beating yourself up for? What are you punishing yourself for?"

Confusedly, I asked, "What do you mean? Am I?"

Chantel told me, "Your injuries are manifesting into the physical because you're mentally beating yourself up so much. It's becoming a cry for attention from your body that this mental and emotional issue needs to be resolved. Your body is literally screaming for help to stop beating it up so much mentally. It's now coming out in the physical. Your emotional and mental pain is becoming physical pain."

That was an eye-opener for me because my whole life I had developed some sort of injury or I was always hurting myself in some way. I had thought I was just accident-prone. Though the more my life was continuing, the more serious these injuries were getting.

There was this underlying issue of me literally mentally beating and abusing myself. I was manifesting it in the physical. I'm grateful this event happened because it's what I have since learned is called a healing crisis. Sometimes things get a bit worse before they can get better.

Sometimes along our healing journey, things do get a little bit shit. You might even get a flu or a cold for a few weeks. That is literally the energy in your body, which is stored as toxins in your body's cells. When you heal, your body detoxes and releases this energy from the cells. It then needs to be let go of through your body, so this is why flu or cold symptoms may arise. It's just previously stored energy coming to the surface to be purged from your body. This is why drinking lots of water is important in the weeks after an energetic healing session.

In my case, I had some deep-rooted issues around believing I deserved to be punished and in pain. Perhaps that's why I had such severe problems manifesting when it came to the car accident recovery. Once we had shifted a few blocks for me, it had come out in the form of a trauma response and a broken arm. In this case, memories from past trauma had been stored in my body's cells and come to the surface of my awareness to be reprocessed.

Also, around this time frame, whilst I had my broken arm in a cast, I was arrested by the police. I was very drunk in the city with a girlfriend. I can't quite fully remember what happened but we ended up separating for the night. I think she went home or left with other people. I stayed because I'd met a couple that I was really getting along with. They were also interested in spirituality and we were having a great time.

Somehow on my drunken walk home to the train station, I ended up getting involved in a police arrest. I think the police were arresting some homeless people and me being the drunken social justice warrior that I thought I had to be, decided to get involved.

They did thank me. The main problem was that because I was drunk, I sometimes don't realise I'm swearing and I accidentally swore at a police officer. They then grabbed my arms to put me under arrest. I had upset and triggered them. They wanted to charge me as well. They grabbed my arm and put it behind me.

Setback

I started screaming.

I was yelling over and over, "Stop. My arm is broken. My arm is broken."

"Get off me, get off me! Get off me!"

I was in so much pain.

I fell to the ground.

I had about six police officers jump on and pin me down on my stomach after that.

Now my hip was also being aggravated.

I ended up being in so much pain my PTSD was set off.

I needed to protect myself—I felt like I was in danger.

That's where I blacked out.

With PTSD, when you're triggered, you're flashed back to a time when you were in danger. In my case, it's usually an instance when my ex was abusing or attacking me. This causes the body to go into fight or flight mode.

When this happens, I think I need to save myself. It doesn't matter if you're my partner that I love. It doesn't matter if you're a police officer and that there are laws. I'm going to black out and protect myself because last time this happened, I nearly died and I'm not going to let that happen again.

Long story short, I was arrested and sent to court in the morning as I had been refused bail. I didn't even realize what I had done until I spoke to the lawyer before we went to court. I was very drunk, which would not have helped the PTSD either. I was so confused. I thought I was just getting done for swearing. I didn't understand why I would get no bail and have to sit in lockup for 12 hours and get taken straight to the courts. Perhaps it was my prior convictions. I was terrified, I thought I was going straight to jail. It didn't help that when I was in lockup, the officers there told me I was likely going to prison from court.

Since this incident, I have come to peace with and accepted things even though the system may be flawed in some ways. For a while, I was terrified of police officers. I do now respect and accept that they're just doing their job and following their training. I do still hope that they're trained to handle mental and physical health scenarios in a more equipped way in the future.

I was in and out of court on bail for roughly three months. I wanted to plead not guilty and fight my case. However, I couldn't afford the legal fees, nor did I want to take the risk that I would be found guilty and then get an even harder sentence.

From what I hear, pleading guilty when you're not actually guilty is quite common for people that go through the legal system. It's easier and the courts treat you better. You get lesser penalties. It becomes a risk-reward thing.

By the end of my court proceedings, I was charged with disorderly conduct in public, obstructing arrest and assaulting an officer. I was informed the officer experienced mild discomfort for the rest of their shift. I'm glad no one was harmed majorly in the incident.

At the time, it felt highly unjust that falling on the ground after my arm in the cast was grabbed was obstructing arrest. It had caused a lot of pain. Then to have a group of officers jump on top of me exacerbating the pain. I was just trying to stop the pain and protect myself. My intention wasn't to hurt anyone. I do forgive and also accept responsibility for my actions though. It's one of the reasons I don't like being too drunk without loving supportive friends around anymore.

One of the more terrifying moments in my life is those months of not knowing if I was going to jail or not. I didn't really tell many people at the time. I was ashamed. I was so hard on myself about it. I thought I was a horrible, bad person. At my final court proceeding, the judge said that I racked up a list of charges in a short timeframe. I had eight in a six-year span. Every charge was alcohol and mental health related. They said to me that my record reflected that I wasn't learning. I wasn't improving. In fact, I was actually getting worse, in the eyes of the law.

In the end, the judge said she was going to give me one more chance. If I kept going down this path, and if I ended up in front of a judge ever again, I would be going to jail. I was in a bit of shock. Though I was also really relieved. I already had in the back of my head that I could quite possibly be going to jail already.

I felt like I had been getting my life back on track from this car accident, even though it wasn't picture-perfect or the healthiest, it was still much better than before. Yet I still needed to change more. I needed to work on myself and really prioritise changing my lifestyle. I also needed to stop being okay with being drunk and alone in the city. I needed to take care of myself. I needed to save myself and keep myself safe. Nobody else was going to do it for me.

Despite it being a pretty crap circumstance, I learnt so much from that experience. I realised if I kept doing the same thing I've always done, I'll get what I have always gotten. Do I want to keep spiralling down? Or do I want to spiral up?

That's when I decided enough was enough. I was sick of my own crap. I couldn't afford to have another rock bottom day like I had prior. Something needed to change and that something was me.

It was not everything around me that needed to change. It was me. I needed to change as that was the only thing I had control over. I needed to stop blaming my external world and take responsibility for myself, my internal world. My subconscious mind was still taking me for a ride. It was time I took back the wheel.

In summary, what I learnt the most from these experiences was that healing was my personal responsibility. Healing you do yourself. Yes, you have a guide or mentor who can teach you or open doors to new ways of being. However, you need to be the one who makes the steps for change. Nobody else is going to do it for you. It's like having a personal trainer to help you lose weight or get fit. They may design a program for you and show you how to exercise but it's you who takes the action that really gets the results.

Healing doesn't go in a straight line. It moves in spirals. Sometimes you come full circle but with a deeper understanding or realisation. It's all a part of the process. Just because you feel like you're going backwards, doesn't mean you are. Sometimes it's three steps forward, two steps back then another three forward. Progress not perfection, as long as you keep moving forward and don't give up, you will get to where you want to be.

Setback

This is the moment I decided I do what really makes me happy in life. I took the leap of faith to follow what I was and still am inspired to do, which is to help others heal in the ways that I had healed. At the time, I mostly wanted to help others with chronic pain not be bedridden by pain anymore. Realising that had the most tremendous impact on me.

Chapter Five

Dragon Magic

"Until you make the unconscious conscious, it will direct your life and you will call it fate."

– Carl Jung

If you understood how powerful your thoughts and words are, you would be careful what you think and speak out loud.

I ended up studying Dragon Magic Hypnotic under Chantel Mary. I loved it. I found something I was super passionate about. For the first time in my life, I found something, other than painting, that I thoroughly enjoyed. I was mostly inspired by Dragon Magic Hypnotic because I had experienced how powerful the results were firsthand. I wanted to be able to make a difference for others too.

Why Dragon Magic Hypnotic?

Dragon Magic is powerful because it focuses on shifting limiting beliefs held in the subconscious mind. According to the first universal Law of Thought, our mind creates our reality through thought. Beliefs (thoughts) are incredibly powerful in shaping our lives. The subconscious part of the mind is heavily responsible for creating our external reality and life experiences.

Our thoughts influence our emotions, which in turn, influence our behaviour. Our emotions can also influence our thoughts, which then impacts how we respond (our behaviour). This takes place in the subconscious mind, which is outside of our conscious awareness.

Using the power of hypnosis and the subconscious mind, your perception of the past can be shifted, resulting in improved feelings of well-being. When operating in an ideal state, the subconscious mind is able to direct the body in healing itself. Dr. Joe Dispenza discusses this subject in depth in his book *Becoming Supernatural*. Hypnosis can assist the mind and body in reconnecting with their natural ability to heal themselves.

Chantel created this form of hypnotherapy based on the downfalls of traditional hypnotherapy as well as the downfalls of kinesiology. She combined what she found were the best parts of the two modalities.

Regular hypnotherapy doesn't really give conscious awareness as to why we have a trigger or limiting belief in the first place. Chantel has mentioned to me that it's more effective to understand why we have a particular issue to begin with in order to overcome it. If we aren't understanding the reason for a certain behaviour, it's still in our unconscious awareness. This means it's more likely to become a reaction to a trigger than a planned action. We become reactive rather than consciously creative in our daily lives.

Kinesiology can take some time for the effects of the healing to take place. Dragon Magic Hypnotic gets faster results in comparison as it works directly with the subconscious mind. Dragon Magic also works well because it's channelled directly from the spiritual world. This makes it more aligned with the person receiving it. It gives more powerful results as it's tailored to cater to individual differences and needs. We are all different after all. We all have different perspectives and experiences. Traditional hypnotherapy scripts are more rigid and may not work for everyone. A channelled Dragon Magic Hypnotic script is more personal and, in my experience, more likely to help as it's different for each person and their own subconscious mind.

Before I explain further, I will give you an interesting finding relating to the subconscious mind, according to Dr. Bruce Lipton[1]. Your thoughts, feelings and reactions in your adult life are most often the same as they were when you were seven. Who you were by age seven is very likely to be who you become as an adult. That is because the blueprint for your subconscious mind is already created by this age.

> *"Whatever we plant in our subconscious mind and nourish with repetition and emotion will one day become a reality."*
> **– Earl Nightingale**

> *"The subconscious mind is ruled by suggestion, it accepts all suggestions – it does not argue with you – it fulfills your wishes."*
> **– Joseph Murphy**

If you find yourself in self-sabotaging patterns, or creating patterns that you don't want in your life, it's likely that your subconscious mind is programmed with limiting beliefs that sustain these undesired patterns.

What Is the Subconscious Mind?

Sigmund Freud[2] first made theories around the conscious and unconscious minds popular in the psychological world. He believed that the mind could be divided into conscious awareness (what we are aware of) and also the unconscious, and subconscious mind (what happens in our mind outside of our awareness).

He theorised that each person's personality is largely outside of their actual awareness. Instead, it's the result of interactions between three parts of the unconscious mind: the id, the ego, and the super-ego. These three components are not connected to any physical brain structure. Though it was theorised they interact and influence what thoughts, ideas and memories actually come into our conscious awareness. Metaphorically speaking, they make up the blueprint or map for how you exist in and make sense of the world, as well as, how you react.

The id exists from birth. It's the thoughts, memories and emotions that are stored in the unconscious mind outside of our awareness. These are instinctive and primal behaviours. For example, an unconscious process outside of our awareness would be inhaling and exhaling air so we can breathe. That isn't something we have to constantly think about doing; it's an automatic behaviour. Breathing can be brought into conscious awareness when you focus on it. However, when you stop focusing on it, your unconscious mind takes over this task again.

The ego evolves from the id. It helps the id meet its survival needs, but in a way that's deemed acceptable and normal by societal standards. It decides what is "morally correct". The ego is influenced by what's external to a person's mind and is heavily impacted by morals. The ego operates in the unconscious, subconscious and conscious minds. It acts as a bridge between having our needs met in a way that supports our morals and beliefs. It's based on upbringing, as well as cultural/societal norms and values. What is deemed acceptable can vary from person to person.

Freud also theorised that the superego begins to crop up at around the age of five. However, it's developing itself prior to then. The super-ego contains all the morals and ideals that we as people learn from our parents or whoever raises us, as well as society as a whole. It's the whole what is right and what is wrong concept. Good old-fashioned values. I'm sure that you've realised by now, we as people seem to have varying definitions of what is right and wrong or what is good and what is bad. This is because we have all had different individual, cultural and historical experiences that have shaped and moulded our subconscious blueprint of what is "good" and what is "bad".

In short, the super-ego encourages us to make ourselves and our behaviour flawless, or our own definition of what that is. Returning to Dr. Lipton's findings, this is based on the experiences we have had mostly up until the age of seven. Experiences, especially trauma, after the age of seven can still impact the subconscious mind, though.

The id, ego and super-ego aren't separate. They are considered to always be coexisting and interacting with one another. These interactions within our mind impact our thoughts, personality and behaviour. Aside from genetics, this is why everybody is different, as everyone has had different experiences influencing how their subconscious mind operates. Everybody has been raised in diverse ways. Everybody is shaped differently, which affects how we respond to what we believe is right and what is wrong.

Imagine your brain being like an antenna for information from your environment, and your subconscious labels it as either "good" or "bad". Whether it's categorised as good or bad depends upon how your blueprint was constructed. How you respond to this categorisation also depends on how your subconscious was wired.

This is also why two people can experience similar situations, however, only one may become traumatised. Trauma occurs from an event that is perceived to be shocking or wrong. An actual trauma doesn't have to take place in order for a person to become traumatised or feel wounded. Only the perception (thought/belief) that something has happened that shouldn't have needs to exist. That is how powerful the mind and its perceptions are.

Conflict easily emerges between these aspects of the unconscious mind. Someone with a more dominant or passive ego may struggle to balance getting their needs met vs following what's morally correct. Someone with a more balanced ego and subconscious mind is better able to work with and overcome these conflicts.

So why am I mentioning this? It's because a lot of our thoughts, feelings and behaviours are influenced by factors outside of our conscious awareness. This is why it's often said that things are easier said than done. Your brain is literally wired for you to respond a certain way, and most of this is determined by the time you're seven!

The subconscious mind also cannot tell the difference between an actual experience and an imagined visualisation. This enables visualisation to be a powerful tool in rewiring how the subconscious operates. This is where the power of hypnosis, Dragon Magic Hypnotic in particular, is able to help rewire your subconscious blueprint so that your mind works with you, and not what seems to be against you.

What Is Dragon Magic Hypnotic?

Dragon Magic Hypnotic is a form of hypnosis that Chantel Mary created based on her understanding of the shortcomings of regular hypnotherapy and kinesiology. Hypnosis involves assisting a person in entering a trance state that's similar to when your brain is asleep. This state is known as a theta-brain wave state. It's a state of deep relaxation where the subconscious mind is more easily altered or re-programmed. This allows a person's expectations to be modified, which then influences how they view the world.

In traditional hypnotherapy, you enter this state by following and visualising along to a script being read, which is designed to shift particular patterns of behaviour, such as smoking cigarettes.

In Dragon Magic Hypnotic, the visualisation, or script, is channelled directly from the spiritual realms. Channelling is when a person has developed their connection with the spiritual world in a way that they can communicate messages on behalf of spiritual beings. A person who acts as a channel is said to be a bridge between the human and spiritual worlds, enabling guidance or messages to be exchanged. The channel also enters a trance-like state as they allow messages to pass through their body from a source outside of them. It's a state of allowing yourself to be used as a physical vessel for messages from spirit to pass through. This skill can be developed by anyone who focuses on growing their spiritual or psychic gifts. We all have the potential to channel.

During a Dragon Magic Hypnotic session, the visualisation is channelled from the spiritual world, making it specifically tailored to whatever your subconscious mind needs to become aware of. You're also able to connect with your spiritual guides and receive guidance. This helped reconnect me with the magical nature of life and the support from the spiritual world.

You're commonly connected with Dragon guides, which is where the Dragon Magic name comes from. We all have a team of spiritual guides and ancestors who are here to help us. I'm sure you've heard the term "guardian angel" before. Well, they're real, it isn't just a saying. We all have these beautiful, spiritual beings looking out for us and guiding us. Whether we listen or see the signs is a different story.

By the end of the session, you've been guided on a meditative journey where your previously limiting beliefs have been replaced by beliefs that are now empowering the subconscious mind.

A limiting belief is simply a belief or thought stored in the subconscious mind that holds us back in life. Limiting beliefs are part of the subconscious roadmap that keeps you stuck. As mentioned previously, a lot of these limiting belief thought patterns are formed in the subconscious mind by the time you're seven years old. These thoughts then go on to influence your personality for the rest of your life or until you put in an effort trying to rewire your subconscious, which can also be done by repeating positive affirmations.

How Is Dragon Magic Hypnotic beneficial?

Dragon Magic Hypnotic is beneficial because, as it's a form of hypnosis, it's able to reprogram the subconscious mind. Dr. Mike Dow, a psychotherapist trained in clinical hypnosis, has stated that due to the theta brain wave state hypnosis encourages, it's able to alter the physical structures of the brain. In a theta brain wave state, the brain is more suggestible in believing it's experiencing something. This means that the visualisations in hypnosis can be likened to an actual experience. The brain cannot tell the difference between what's real and what's visualised.

By creating positive, safe spaces through Dragon Magic Hypnotic's visualisations, a person is able to overcome repetitive situations or feelings that previously held them back in life. This is hugely beneficial, especially in regard to trauma. Trauma alters brain structure so that a person is more prepared for the potential threat of danger occurring. In other words, a person who has experienced trauma usually has a heightened fight or flight response.

The fight or flight response is helpful when it comes to protecting us from the immediate threat of danger, like if a tiger was hunting you in the wild. However, a traumatised person's fight or flight response is more easily set off. This results in challenging reactions from the individual, such as extreme anxiety, panic attacks or literally lashing out at perceived danger, even if there's no real danger.

After domestic violence, I had PTSD and was very easily triggered by what I perceived to be a threat to my safety. If a person used a tone that was slightly off, I would start shaking and sweating, as I believed my life was at risk. My mind would revisit past traumas. I wouldn't be able to tell the difference between the reality in front of me, and the reality of my past. This made personal relationships quite challenging. I did push a lot of people away because of my perceptions and inappropriate responses. I also was quite socially anxious as it felt like I couldn't really trust anyone.

Not to mention, throwing the after-effects of the car accident into the mix, I was highly stressed and ill trusting of the world in general. I was surviving to get by each day. I thought that it was me vs the world. When really it was me vs my subconscious mind.

By receiving Dragon Magic Hypnotic as a treatment, I was able to shift limiting beliefs programmed into my subconscious such as, "The world is unsafe," or, "People are out to hurt me," into empowering beliefs such as, "I'm safe and supported," and, "It's safe to trust other people."

It sounds small, but having subconscious beliefs around the world being an unsafe place and that people were going to harm me was creating a life that I felt I had to escape from. One where I was always looking over my shoulder or waiting for the next person to try to take advantage of or hurt me. Shifting these beliefs enabled me to shift my perspective to where I no longer viewed the world as a bad and dangerous place. I was no longer waiting for the next traumatic incident to happen. I was able to relax and not be on edge. Panic attacks weren't so easily triggered.

I also started attracting genuine, loving friendships into my life. As I shifted my subconscious belief that people were dangerous, I was no longer feeling drawn to dangerous people. I actually started to be able to see them for who they were so I could distance myself. Due to shifting my beliefs, I was also able to be a better friend, which led to people being better friends to me. It's really interesting how beliefs in the subconscious mind can play out in reality like this.

Another way Dragon Magic Hypnotic is beneficial is because the visualisation is channelled straight from the spiritual realms. This means that it's more personalised and accounts for differences in people's subconscious minds. Our subconsciouses are all programmed differently after all. Some people may need to hear something worded a particular way in order for it to make sense to their subconscious so that a shift in beliefs can occur.

From receiving Dragon Magic Hypnotic treatments, I was able to overcome chronic pain that was leaving me exhausted and bedridden, especially after work shifts. Prior to that, I struggled to make it downstairs to my apartment's basement to get my art supplies out if I wanted to paint. After multiple sessions over time, I was not only able to work longer hours on my feet but I was also signed back up at the gym and doing workouts! This was something that I thought would be impossible to do again.

During the treatment process, it was uncovered that I had limiting beliefs in my subconscious about thinking I was a bad person, as well as that I deserved to be punished. This pattern had been playing out in my life consistently, from the crappy partners I would choose, to the point where I kept manifesting these awful injuries and was physically in pain. Remember that the subconscious mind exists mostly outside of our awareness. Consciously, I may have thought a certain partner was good for me. This is because subconsciously I thought they were good for me as they were confirming my already limiting beliefs. The subconscious mind doesn't discriminate, it just plays out its blueprint or programming.

It wasn't until after Dragon Magic Hypnotic, that I realised how much I would mentally beat myself up. I used to have horrible thoughts circling around my head that I just couldn't seem to shake. This was something I had experienced my entire life and I thought was normal. I just couldn't seem to stop being so hard on myself or thinking I deserved bad things to happen to me. I had this innate belief there was something significantly wrong with me and I needed to always be better than what I was. I have since been able to shift these beliefs into ones such as, "I'm more than enough" and, "I deserve good things to happen to me."

Dragon Magic Hypnotic really helped me remove those negative thought patterns that I had struggled with my whole life. Treatment from Dragon Magic also enabled me to overcome the slowed processing I had been living with since hitting my head. My mind went from a place of confusion that was torturing me to becoming my happy sanctuary. I'm a big believer that heaven and hell exist within your mind. I was living in hell in my mind for so many years due to the traumas I had been through. I was stuck in these repeating patterns of behaviour that I just couldn't seem to break free from. My fate had felt like a life of tragedy until my limiting beliefs were shifted.

I honestly now believe that my mind is heaven. It's paradise. I would not call it perfect as stuff still crops up every now and then, but I can quiet that little chatter. I can comfort and nurture myself. I can love it for what it is and accept it. It doesn't control me. It doesn't rule my life. My subconscious mind doesn't take me on that same bloody ride. I'm no longer living to survive each day. I'm living to thrive. My life has unfolded into one I never expected. I honestly thought I was doomed to a life of pain and suffering, waiting for the next traumatic event to occur.

Many people have questions or concerns about hypnosis, such as:

You may be concerned about hypnosis and whether it's a form of mind control.

I understand that the entertainment world has made it appear that way. However, it isn't what most people think. You're only in a trance that is a focused state of relaxation, you're aware and present the whole time. You can snap yourself out of the trance at any time if you feel uncomfortable. You're in control of yourself the entire time.

You may have also tried it or heard of somebody who has tried it, and it didn't work for them.

This is because the mind and beliefs are powerful. People who are more open to suggestions are more likely to be successfully hypnotised. If you don't believe it works, then it isn't going to work. It's like watching a horror movie and telling yourself it's fake or not real. The movie will appear less scary than if you immersed yourself fully into the experience as if it were a true story.

You may not be sure about the channelling and spiritual side of it.

I understand it can seem daunting if you haven't experienced it before or understand little about it. My best suggestion would be to keep an open mind if you feel comfortable. Otherwise, you don't have to try it, traditional hypnotherapy and hypnosis can be just as effective. I'm simply sharing a form of hypnotherapy that I'm familiar with and that has helped me significantly.

Challenge Your Limiting Beliefs

Firstly, you could practice becoming aware of your thoughts. See if you can simply observe them without reacting to or judging them. I think understanding that you aren't actually your thoughts and that you're the observer of your thoughts is quite powerful in taking back control of your mind. You don't have to listen to or identify with every thought that enters your mind. Separating yourself from your thoughts can take practice. Meditation practices do help with this.

As you become consciously aware of the thoughts you tell yourself, make note of them. Which thoughts are limiting and negative? Which thoughts are empowering? Keep the empowering thoughts and repeat them as affirmations to strengthen them within your subconscious mind. See if you can flip the limiting thoughts into positive ones such as, "I can't afford that" into, "This isn't a financial priority for me right now." Or, "I'm ugly," to, "I'm absolutely beautiful."

So those negative thoughts you made note of? Those are some of your limiting beliefs! You can work on flipping these beliefs in your subconscious mind by turning them into positive affirmations. The best time to do this is within the first hour of waking up, as your brain is still in a theta-wave dream state from sleeping. This means the subconscious is more easily altered at this time.

Summary

The mind and its thoughts are incredibly powerful. Your thoughts (beliefs) have an impact on your perception and reality.

The subconscious mind stores ideas or beliefs which play out as repetitive patterns of behaviour in your life. Some of these beliefs are limiting and hold us back in life or create suffering.

Dragon Magic Hypnotic is a form of hypnotherapy that allows limiting beliefs to be replaced by empowering ones, using channelled visualisations from the spiritual realms.

Dragon Magic Hypnotic really helped me gain confidence and the ability to believe in myself again after suffering from the impacts of significant life traumas. I was able to turn my pain into passion for life. I was no longer bedridden from chronic pain.

I would highly recommend observing the thoughts that pass through your mind during the day and making a note of them. See if you can flip any of them into positives, and then say them out loud as affirmations.

Upon completing Dragon Magic Hypnotic, I started seeing clients. I was excited to be able to help people create change in their life, such as overcoming obstacles at work or difficulties in their relationships.

However, after a few months, I felt like I wanted to be able to offer another modality to people. One technique may be very effective for one person, but another may be more beneficial for another person.

So, I continued my wellness journey, learning more modalities in order to expand the ways that I could help myself and others improve our quality of life.

Chapter Six

Reiki Hands

"Give yourself permission to let it hurt, but also allow yourself the permission to let it heal."
— **Nikki Rowe**

Have you ever wondered how Jesus actually performed the healing miracles that he did? If you don't believe in Jesus then this can be hypothetical. How can somebody possibly heal these people? With their hands? What energy was being tapped into?

Why Reiki?

Let's begin with why Reiki (*Ray-key*) is beneficial. Reiki promotes deep feelings of relaxation and acceptance. It helps with easing negative thoughts, as well as puts the brain into a relaxing trance state, similar to when you sleep at night or are receiving hypnosis.

Reiki is great if you're not comfortable discussing your thoughts and feelings. It's also good if you're not even aware of what the next step you need to take is.

I also enjoy Reiki because it's safe and relaxing. It can be given either with hands on or off the body. The non-invasiveness of this treatment is especially beneficial for people who have trauma, particularly around being touched.

It's considered a gentle approach because it only shifts what you're ready to shift. It works best when the energy is allowed to direct itself without any control of where in your body it should go.

Reiki is also beneficial because it's timeless. You can send Reiki energy into the past, present, as well as future. For instance, if you're anxious about an upcoming event or meeting, you could send Reiki into that future situation to help ease your anxiety.

Did you know that in some Eastern practices, it's believed everyone has a system of chakras, or energy centres, that exist within their body or energetic field? When these chakras are imbalanced, undesirable states of being, such as physical or mental ailments, are more likely to occur. When they're balanced, these things are less likely to manifest as your energy flow is aligned.

> *"Disease is often an accumulation of dammed-up energy. When we learn how energy moves through the chakras, we can begin to allow it to flow freely through our bodies, creating greater health."*
>
> **– Deepak Chopra**

"Opening your chakras and allowing cosmic energies to flow through your body will ultimately refresh your spirit and empower your life."

– Barbara Marciniak

Reiki helps to balance this chakra system. Having under or overactive chakras can send you and your body into a state of disease or disharmony.

What Is Reiki?

Reiki is simply pure love energy. Its energy is very relaxing and helps you feel a greater level of acceptance in life. In Japanese, Reiki is translated as *"Rei"* meaning sacred and spirit, and as *"ki"* or *"qi"*, which you may be already familiar with. Qi is popular in Chinese or Eastern-based health medicines and is known as a universal lifeforce energy. The energy that lives in everything, including inanimate objects, such as this book.

In Chinese medicine, it's believed that when a person's qi or life force energy is unbalanced or disrupted, then they suffer from poor health and disease. A healthy person would have balanced qi energy.

There are different forms of Reiki across the world. It has since been discovered that it was forgotten ancient knowledge and was used throughout different societies, including the ancient Egyptians. The system that I was trained in originated in Japan and is called Usui Reiki Ryoho.

This form of Reiki was developed by Master Mikao Usui (1865-1926). Usui searched for the answer to the question I asked at the beginning of this chapter. He wanted to understand how people like Jesus and the Buddha were able to heal people.

After travelling the world, he eventually decided to meditate and fast from food for 21 days on a sacred mountain. On the last day, a bright white light struck Usui where he received an understanding of Reiki. He felt replenished despite his fasting and excitedly raced down the mountain. He hurt his foot so he grabbed it with his hand. He was amazed to find the bleeding and pain stopped. He was healed.

Later, he healed a couple of others. He had uncovered the healing power he had been on a quest to find. This inspired Usui to start schools where he taught this modality and it has been passed on since.

Reiki is given by the practitioner placing their hands on or above energy centres on a person's body. Reiki energy is channelled from the universe, through the top of the practitioner's head and out through the palms of their hands. Reiki works to balance these energy centres.

Reiki is a holistic therapy because it works on balancing your four energetic bodies, which are said to make up a person's entire being. These four bodies interrelate with one another and are known as the physical, emotional, mental and spiritual bodies.

Rather than looking at segmented parts of you that need treatment, Reiki works on you as the whole picture of you.

Reiki works on the physical body by assisting your body's own ability to heal and repair itself. It can cleanse the body of toxins. It also works with your consciousness to help grow a higher awareness of what your body needs, like correct nutrition or exercise.

Reiki works on the mental body by providing relief around your thinking processes. It can help with negative thinking and provide a deep state of relaxation. Reiki can also help provide deeper insight and awareness of self, which can lead to a better understanding of your potential and skills in life.

Reiki works on the emotional body by flowing into all aspects of your emotions, including those you may have repressed. It also encourages feeling and being more loving, caring, trusting and friendly. It helps with forgiveness and letting go of past hurt.

Finally, Reiki works on the spiritual body by being absorbed into your entire energetic field, or aura. This helps you with self-love and acceptance, letting go of judgments, and being more understanding of the world. Reiki can assist you in pursuing your individual path toward developing your spirituality and feeling connected with the divine, source energy or God, whichever term you'd like to use. It's practically all the same essence, just a different label.

It's also important to highlight that Reiki isn't a cure, it's a facilitator of healing. By receiving Reiki, the space for healing to take place is created, however, it's up to the individual to take the actions to improve their health. You could say that a Reiki practitioner opens the door for health benefits, but it's the client or person receiving the Reiki that actually takes the steps.

What Are Chakras?

As well as these four bodies, Reiki helps support a balanced flow of energy across your chakra system. For this book, I will only focus on the seven main chakras, however, there are many more chakras within your body.

Chakra is a Sanskrit word for "wheel" or "disc". They can be described as the energy centres that exist within you that act like filters for the energies that enter and exit your body. They're cone-shaped in appearance. Please refer to the diagram to see where they're located in the body. Feel free to colour them yourself if you wish to.

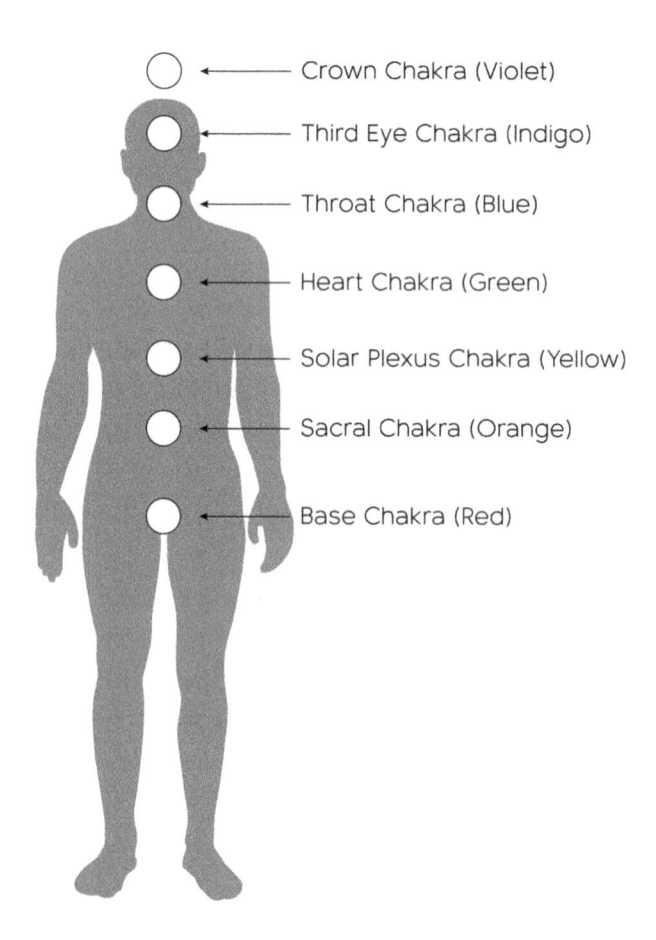

- Crown Chakra (Violet)
- Third Eye Chakra (Indigo)
- Throat Chakra (Blue)
- Heart Chakra (Green)
- Solar Plexus Chakra (Yellow)
- Sacral Chakra (Orange)
- Base Chakra (Red)

The first chakra is known as the base or root chakra. This chakra is connected to the physical body and the colour red. It relates to survival needs and feelings of security. Issues around your home, physical body, job and finances are commonly associated with this chakra.

The second chakra, the sacral, is also connected to the physical body, but with respect to physical sensations, creativity and sexuality. Issues around shock, trauma, sexual intimacy and pleasure relate to this chakra. The sacral chakra is orange.

The third chakra, the solar plexus, is yellow and connected to the emotional body. It's said that issues regarding the ego relate to the solar plexus. Problems relating to self-esteem, control, personal freedom and addiction are associated.

The next is the heart chakra, which is also connected with the emotional body. The heart chakra is connected to the colour green. The heart chakra is all about unconditional love and being able to give as well as receive it. It's also associated with personal boundaries.

The next chakra is your throat chakra, which is connected to the colour blue. It relates to your ability to communicate and express yourself authentically and honestly. It also relates to whether you speak your truth or not.

The third eye chakra is located in the middle of your forehead, above your brows, and is connected to the colour indigo. This chakra is connected with the pineal gland in the brain and is involved with psychic and intuitive abilities and your thought processes. It's connected to the mind.

The seventh chakra is your crown chakra and is associated with the colour violet or purple. Your crown chakra is just above your head in your aura or energetic field. It's what connects you to the divine light and the cosmos and energies from above. The crown chakra helps us see and feel the connection of everything and everyone in unity. The "allness" of life, as we recognise that everything is connected in some way.

When out of balance, these chakras can be overactive or underactive. In the following table, I have compared what it can mean when these chakras are balanced and imbalanced.

Chakra	Balanced	Blocked	Overactive
Base/Root	Feeling safe and secure in regard to survival needs, feelings of stability and peace, feeling connected and grounded in reality	Low energy, poor concentration, feeling isolated, financial stress, feeling disconnected, ungroundedness, fearfulness	Feeling like survival needs aren't met. Anxiety, stress, fearfulness, aggression
Sacral	Experiencing pleasures in life with balance, feeling joyful, feeling present in the moment, openness	Decreased libido, decreased creativity, lack of joy and pleasure, fears around intimacy	Addictive or over-indulgent behaviour, feeling traumatised, emotional overreactions, restlessness, co-dependency
Solar Plexus	Confidence in wisdom and authentic power, honesty, respect of self	Feelings of insecurity & inferiority, indecisiveness, confusion, passive aggressiveness, neediness or timidness, powerlessness	Irritable, controlling, greed, lack of empathy or compassion for others, domineering, perfectionism
Heart	Truly able to give and receive love, healthy boundaries	Heartbroken, difficulty trusting, feeling disconnected from the body, circulation issues, bitterness	Lack of boundaries, over gives, self-sacrificing, jealousy, co-dependency, heart palpitations, heartburn
Throat	Able to speak with clarity from a place of truth and love, easy to express self through written and oral communication, diplomatic	Shyness, quiet, inability to express feelings, thoughts and truths secretive, feeling misunderstood	Interrupts others, difficulty listening, overexaggerates, gossips, cruel words, lies, feel unheard, throat issues, mouth ulcers, dental problems
Third Eye	Feel connected with both spiritual and physical worlds, imaginative, clear thinking	Feeling disconnected from spirituality or higher power, fatigue, headaches, sinus issues, overly sceptical, poor focus	Difficulty relating to being human, overly distracted by the spiritual realm, nightmares, hallucinations
Crown	Buddhist teaching "Nirvana" state, overcome suffering, feeling at one with all of creation	Best to focus on balancing the other six chakras to balance the crown	Best to focus on balancing the other six chakras to balance the crown

How Is Reiki Beneficial?

Personally, I've found that Reiki helped me reach a greater level of self-acceptance and acceptance of life and it helped me feel more relaxed and supported. It has also assisted me in gaining trust in the universe and life around me. It's really helped me with balancing my chakra system as I had quite a few things blocked or out of whack, which most people do.

I also used to suffer from quite bad insomnia and racing thoughts. I found Reiki really beneficial in helping with both of these things. It also helped me connect with and find my inner purpose.

I had a really cool instance of doing Reiki on another person recently. They had torn their calf muscle and had been told it would be a six-week recovery period involving physio. As we were in two separate locations, I did two distant Reiki sessions, about a week apart. Within three weeks, the physio was amazed at how quickly their body had regenerated and recovered. They were discharged from physio halfway through the initial recovery plan. I was told by the person that they were certain it was thanks to the Reiki healing I had done. I think this story is a really good example of how powerful and special this modality is, even without being physically present.

I also did Reiki on myself after recent surgery on my arm. My arm had difficulties healing well in the past, hence I managed to re-break it so easily years later. In the past, I had experienced quite a few complications with surgeries and recoveries. This was my smoothest recovery ever. There were no delays or setbacks. My doctors even told me that my arm had healed beautifully.

I thank Reiki for that as it helped me have acceptance over another surgery, despite the triggers I've had in the past around hospitals.

It also helped alleviate any anxiety and stress that would have consumed me in the past.

So, you may be saying it's all a scam. This stuff isn't real, this seems farfetched. It all sounds a bit made up to me.

I understand that, as with any industry, there can be fakes and frauds that give things a bad name. I'd also suggest not knocking it until you try it. It's just one of those things, you just don't know until you try it.

You may have also had one session before and felt nothing. I understand that.

One session probably isn't going to result in any noticeable differences in all honesty. It depends on how imbalanced your chakras are or the state of the blockages in your energetic field. I normally recommend at least four to five sessions before you might really start to feel an impact.

Balance Your Chakras

Although I endorse receiving Reiki if it's something you feel interested in, it's not essential to balance your chakras. There are many different ways you can work on your chakra system.

I would suggest going back to the table in this chapter to decide which chakra you may want to start working on, based on symptoms you may relate to. The following are some examples which you may like to try.

For balancing all of the chakras, you can look up sound frequencies such as binaural beats or meditation tracks. I normally find plenty of these for free on YouTube. Each chakra can be balanced using a corresponding sound frequency, or even mantra.

Other useful activities for balancing and developing your chakras are meditation, breathwork and yoga. I will discuss meditation in more detail later in its own chapter. Breathwork is a type of meditation that is more active as it focuses on using breathing techniques that are based on yoga practices. Many people find breathwork helpful if slowing their thinking process is too difficult in standard meditation.

In regards to yoga, there are many different forms—some more spiritual than others. I think no matter what type of yoga you do, moving your physical body and stretching are going to be beneficial either way. Of course, doing a more spiritual-based yoga practice is going to develop your chakras quicker. There are specific yoga positions that can be held that focus on a particular chakra.

I will now give a few dot points for each chakra specifically.

Balancing the root chakra activities:

- Walking barefoot on the Earth's surface, such as beach sand or grass
- Using red, black or earthy-toned crystals, such as red jasper, black tourmaline, garnet and hematite
- Doing activities that connect you with the Earth, such as hiking, gardening, or swimming at the beach
- Wearing the colour red or green
- Eating foods that are red in colour
- Affirmations such as, "I'm safe", "I'm supported", or "I belong"

Balancing the sacral chakra activities:

- Journalling your feelings
- Using orange crystals, such as carnelian, orange citrine and tiger eye
- Doing activities that are creative, including cooking
- Practicing stillness—even if it's only one minute to start with
- Making peace with the past or therapy for past trauma
- Wearing the colours orange or turquoise
- Eating foods that are orange in colour
- Affirmations such as, "I'm allowed to feel joy", "I embrace my sexuality" or "I'm worthy"

Balancing the solar plexus chakra activities:

- Practicing body postures that show confidence, such as standing straight and confidently with your shoulders back
- Using yellow or gold crystals such as yellow citrine, pyrite, and lemon quartz
- Making peace with the past or therapy for past trauma
- Doing things that make you happy or feel confident
- Wearing the colours yellow or blue
- Eating foods that are yellow in colour
- Affirmations such as, "I feel capable", "I'm able to assert myself with confidence" or "I surrender control"

Balancing the heart chakra activities:

- Spending time with loved ones, including pets
- Using green or pink crystals, such as rose quartz, rhodonite and green aventurine
- Establishing or maintaining clear boundaries with others
- Hugging people more often
- Allowing yourself to feel emotions rather than push them aside
- Spending time in nature with lots of green scenery
- Eating foods that are green in colour
- Wearing the colours green or pink
- Affirmations such as, "I'm lovable", "I have gratitude", "I listen to my heart" or "I'm open"

Balancing the throat chakra activities:

- Singing or humming so that sound vibrates from your throat
- Using blue crystals, such as turquoise, aquamarine and blue lace agate
- Doing stretches for your neck muscles
- Practicing honesty
- Journalling your thoughts
- Wearing the colour blue
- Affirmations such as, "I speak my truth with ease", "I express how I feel" or "It's safe to be honest"

Balancing the third eye chakra activities:

- Meditating
- Using crystals, such as lapus lazuli, moonstone or amethyst
- Getting enough good quality sleep
- Reducing toxins in the diet
- Drinking clean, spring water free from fluoride
- Wearing the colour indigo
- Affirmations such as, "I trust my intuition", "I see and think clearly" or "I'm present in the now"

Balancing the crown chakra activities:

- Meditation or yoga
- Using crystals such as clear quartz or amethyst
- Spending time in nature observing the beauty surrounding you
- Wearing the colour violet or purple
- Affirmations such as, "I honour the divine within me" or "I'm open to divine wisdom"

Chapter Seven

Reiki Master

"Reiki can never and will never belong to just one person or one organisation. Reiki is the spiritual heritage of all humanity."

– Dr. Mikao Usui

After being trained in Reiki 1, I fell in love with the modality.

I decided to pursue Reiki 2 and then a master's. It seemed like a no-brainer to be able to pass on this beautiful form of therapy. I also felt inspired to continue Usui's legacy. This is why I thought I would dedicate a chapter specifically to why I became a Reiki Master.

There are three levels of Reiki you can be trained in. Level 1 introduces you to the Reiki frequency. Level 2 you're qualified as a practitioner. After completing your master's, you can train others.

I'm so passionate about Reiki that I really do believe it would be awesome if the whole world was attuned to this beautiful frequency. Especially because it's literally just pure, unconditional love energy.

Why Be Attuned to Reiki?

I think that most people would gain from being attuned to at least Reiki level one for a number of reasons.

The first is in relation to Usui's legacy. His goal when he started his schools was to help people improve their own health and well-being, especially if they couldn't afford medical care. Usui wanted Reiki to be passed on so that more people can help their own health. I think Usui's vision is still very relevant today, if not more, with long waitlists or expensive healthcare that not everybody has access to.

Another reason is that I think it's important to have knowledge and awareness about the energetic bodies and chakra system, as well as how to cleanse and develop yours. A widespread understanding would take pressure off of health systems, whilst improving societal health and well-being. Of course, there are other ways that this can be done. However, in my experience, Reiki is a simple introduction and yet quite effective.

I also think being attuned is beneficial because it's pure love energy. I find it so beautiful to connect with the frequency of Reiki and be able to share it. There's something otherworldly about it. It does help you realise there's some power greater than our human existence out there and it loves and wants the best for us.

I do believe it'd be helpful for more people to be attuned to Reiki throughout the world. It's the whole ripple effect concept. When you heal yourself, it flows out into the environment around you. Then you also indirectly heal the people around you, which ripples throughout their environment, and so on. The possibilities with how to use Reiki are endless. You can give Reiki to anything, including food, water, pets and plants!

So, hypothetically, if everybody had this Reiki knowledge, and we were taking responsibility for healing ourselves and the planet, how cool would that be? I think it really could help make the world a better place. Not to mention the beautiful, amazing impact on the individual self alone.

Furthermore, I have found being Reiki-attuned is beneficial as it helps with hangovers. Yep, it helps with hangovers!

I believe that the goal of wellness or healthcare sessions should be to treat the client holistically and assist them in helping themselves with confidence. I think supporting somebody in gaining autonomy over their health, well-being and quality of life is incredibly impactful.

> *"The teacher who is indeed wise does not bid you to enter the house of his wisdom but rather leads you to the threshold of your mind."*
> **– Kahlil Gibran**

> *"Your Reiki power is like an aura, it's a glow, and you're radiating out... no darkness can penetrate you."*
> **– Hawayo Takata.**

It doesn't matter if you're seeing a traditional or an alternative practitioner. Ideally, you don't want to be largely dependent on someone or something. That can get expensive and contribute to a lack of confidence in yourself and your health. Are you really improving?

What Is a Reiki Attunement?

A Reiki attunement or being Reiki attuned means being "tuned" into the Reiki frequency. Imagine it being like Reiki is a radio channel and you're a radio. The process of receiving a Reiki attunement is similar to a radio being tuned into a specific radio station's frequency so it can play its channel. In other words, it's simply just tuning your body to be able to give and receive the frequency of Reiki.

Once you have been attuned to the Reiki frequency, it stays with you for life. If you stop practicing and using Reiki, you may feel disconnected from it and as if you've lost the Reiki. You haven't and don't need to be re-attuned. It's just like building muscle at the gym, it may waste away, but it can be built back with repeated use. You just simply need to trust it and it will flow.

How Is Being Attuned to Reiki Beneficial?

Reiki works holistically on the body because it's amazing at balancing your chakra systems and the four energetic bodies. This is how Reiki has a large array of health and quality of life benefits. For this reason, I would highly recommend anybody who's interested to get attuned to Reiki. It can benefit you across all domains of your life, as it will shift whatever needs shifting within your chakra and energy body systems.

It's terrific because you can use it to cleanse your own energy field from blockages that may be present. We all get blockages in our energetic field and it's beneficial to clear them before they manifest into a state of disharmony or disease, which I will be discussing more in the Crystals and Metaphysics chapter.

Reiki generally helps you feel super relaxed and a lot of us in society are stressed—whether we're traumatized or not. Imagine being able to do Reiki on yourself instead of relying on Valium or marijuana to calm down. Of course, there's nothing wrong with the latter two either—no judgment. We all have our preferences.

In her book, *Dodging Energy Vampires*, Christiane Northrup M.D.[3] discusses how highly sensitive people (commonly termed empaths) get better results with metaphysical-based treatments than medical ones. Highly sensitive people are given this label because they're more impacted by denser energies. I'm one of those people who's negatively impacted by medications. If meds agree with you—that's fantastic too! I'm not saying stop taking your meds and get attuned to Reiki. I'm just suggesting alternatives that really advanced my well-being.

Being attuned personally helped me enormously with being an insomniac. I used to toss and turn with an overactive racing mind most nights, reliant on cannabis. Nowadays, I can give myself Reiki before bed and the deep relaxation it promotes helps me drift away to sleep.

Since my experiences with Reiki, I have come to learn how sacred this modality really is. There's something mystical and powerful about it. It opens doors to a world of energy that's frequently undetected by many of us. This has helped me feel more connected with life and as if I belong in this world.

Reiki can also be sent to help situations. If there's a conflict happening, you can send Reiki into that situation and the highest and greatest good will be encouraged. It might not defuse the fight because maybe that argument needs to play out that way. If you send some, the worst that happens is that person's energy field (aura) rejects it and it bounces. You can't force it on somebody. They have to be open to receiving it, either consciously or subconsciously. Although it's best to ask permission first.

Another thing that being attuned to Reiki was able to change the game for was me looking after houseplants. I was notorious for killing them. Since being attuned to Reiki, I magically have a green thumb and my plants thrive! I've even brought a few back from the brink of death.

I'm sure this benefit would be a lot of people's favourite. If you have a hangover, you simply just do Reiki on your head if you've got a headache or on your stomach if it's upset. I have done Reiki on my stomach after a big night of drinking. I literally threw up within 10 minutes of giving myself Reiki. I thought, *oh my god that made me worse!* Then I realized, that alcohol must have been sitting in my stomach from the night before. The Reiki was pushing it out of my body by vomiting. The easiest and fastest way to excrete a swallowed toxin.

So, you may be thinking what if it does something that shocks me?

Reiki is pure love. It can't harm. It only does what it's ready to do. So, an example of this would be when I first started with Reiki. I was smoking pot regularly. Not heavily like in prior years, but I was still using it more than I felt was okay.

It wasn't until months and months along my Reiki journey, that I actually just woke up one day and was like, "You know what, I don't want to do this daily anymore."

The shift slowly, gently, and gradually happened. Almost like it had happened overnight. I just woke up different one day. I can't even tell you what exactly shifted to help me stop being reliant. That's what I mean by Reiki is a subtle and gentle approach that only does what a person is ready for.

It only does the highest and greatest good for yourself and all on the planet. So, if it doesn't align with that, which you could call the divine plan, then it's not really going to do much. You can't use Reiki to manipulate or control anything.

You might still be thinking this is all made up.

That's okay. You don't have to accept this at all. This is just my story and my experience and what has helped me. What helps me might not help you. You don't have to accept what I'm saying.

You could also be thinking that this is all a placebo effect.

Well, technically everything is a placebo effect if you break it down. The power of the mind is so strong, we can use our thoughts to influence and create the reality around us. So yes, the placebo effect could be happening because if you believe something to be true, then it's most likely going to happen!

This is why scientific experiments use a control group. Even scientists know that the mind and the power of belief are powerful. This is how somebody can take a sugar pill posed as medicine, and say they feel as if their symptoms have improved from it. The symptoms get better because that is how powerful your mind and thoughts are!

Connecting with Energies

I recommend researching more into Reiki if you're feeling drawn to it. Amongst the Reiki community, there's a saying that you don't find Reiki, it finds you. When you're ready to experience what Reiki has to offer, you will feel curious about connecting with it.

If you're interested, I would definitely suggest finding someone you feel aligned with to attune you. You're welcome to contact me as I do run courses from time to time. At the back of the book is a discounted special offer to my readers, if you're wanting to learn Reiki.

I also suggest practicing feeling variances in energies. A simple practical exercise you can do is find various animate and inanimate objects, such as a houseplant and a glass cup. Slow things down and tune into your breath by taking deep, slow breaths, in and out. Rub your palms together so that friction builds. Then, one at a time, place your hands just above each item without directly touching it. Pay attention to what you notice. See if you can feel a difference in energies emanating from each item.

This may take more practice for some than others. Everyone is different. However, everyone has the ability to feel energy. Different energies feel unalike. With practice, you definitely can feel a difference in the energies coming off of different items, animals, people or even buildings in this world.

At first, the energetic differences may be subtle, but with more practice, your ability to detect these differences should strengthen.

Chapter Eight

Colour Mirrors

"The whole point is to live life and be – to use all the colours in the crayon box."

– RuPaul

Dragon Magic Hypnotic helped me replace limiting beliefs with empowering beliefs so that I could transform my life situation and break repetitive cycles. Reiki opened the doorway to holistic health, as well as unblocking and balancing my chakras. The colour mirrors system completely changed the game.

It contributed to another significant leap in my personal growth. Upon first seeing the coloured bottles, I found them so fascinating. I was drawn to them. I needed to learn more, and so I did.

Why the Colour Mirrors System?

The colour mirrors system unveils colour, as the mirror of our internal world that's reflected in our external reality. Remember that our subconscious mind reflects our experience of the world external to us. Well, colour and the subconscious mind play a role together too. Information stored in the subconscious can also be explored and transformed using this system.

This modality guides you in exploring deeper insights about yourself and life itself. It's a soft and gentle approach toward facing trauma or life difficulties, which may otherwise be quite heavy to process and overcome.

This system propelled my life forward in refreshing ways I could never have imagined. I have had major realisations and shifts occur since working with the system. My whole perspective on myself, life and reality has changed. It really is a transformational system when experienced.

This system reawakens you to the fun and magic of colour and life. It re-connected me with the playful nature of my inner child. The magnificent colours and energies oozing from the bottles made facing the darker aspects and experiences of myself, and my past, quite an enlighteningly light-hearted experience.

Colour Mirrors Therapy provided answers to difficulties I was experiencing in a gentle and loving way, without having to revisit the traumatic event. This allowed me to let go of the remaining shame and guilt I had been carrying. I was also able to come to a place of peace and acceptance of myself and life, even with issues I hadn't realised I had prior.

Do you remember back to school, the science or physics lesson where we played around with the glass, mirrors and light? The one where we saw how colour exists on a spectrum of light that's like a rainbow when fragmented. Well, the reason I'm mentioning it is because colour is simply light energy. Everything visible to the eye consists of light energy. Even your body is made up of light. It has a form that absorbs and reflects frequencies of light, which is what becomes the colour we see.

"What do we call visible light? We call it colour. But the electromagnetic spectrum runs to zero in one direction and infinity in the other, so really, children, mathematically, all of light is invisible."

– Anthony Doerr

"Your attitude is like a box of crayons that colour your world. Constantly colour your picture grey, and your picture will always be bleak. Try adding some bright colours to the picture by including humour, and your picture begins to lighten up."

– Allen Klein

I understand the idea of using colours to overcome trauma and improve quality of life may seem a bit farfetched. However, living in a state of denial and avoidance only keeps you stuck. I have found that to be more painful than trying something new. Even if that new thing does not make logical sense at the time.

What Is Colour?

Going back to that science lesson I mentioned earlier, various waves and particles of light are emitted from the sun and reach the Earth. Light energy exists as a spectrum, with each colour having a certain frequency along that spectrum. This is similar to sound energy and how different sounds have different energetic frequencies along their spectrum. Light and sound are really just two different spectrums of types of energy.

Depending on the properties of something on Earth or in the universe, particular frequencies of light are absorbed and the rest of the light is reflected back into the external world. The colours in the spectrum of light that are reflected, become the colours that our eyes see. Seeing colour is similar to how the brain recognises and interprets symbols. The interpretation of colour can be likened to being a language that the brain interprets outside of our conscious awareness. Colour, or light, helps us to understand and interact with the surrounding world on an unconscious and subconscious level. It's one of the languages of the soul, like music.

What Are Colour Mirrors?

The colour mirrors system was first channelled by Melissie Jolly in South Africa in 2001. This system uses the different energies of each colour frequency, in the form of bottles of oils and essences that have undergone a special creation process. This mysterious process is what adds to their unique magical qualities. Pictured next are examples of what some of the bottles and essences in the system look like.

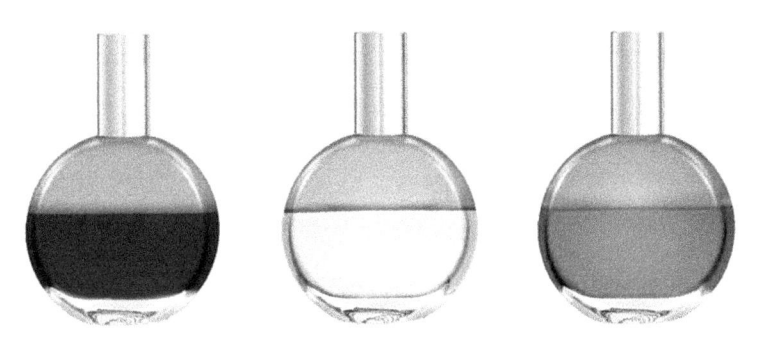

In explaining how this system works, Melissie Jolly and Korani Connolly[4] state, "The system takes the energies of light and uses them to address deeply buried thoughts and beliefs that reside within your cells," and, "Colour Mirrors transmits the voice of love not just to your mind, but to the cells of your body. When your cells receive a message – any message – they log the information. They have an innate intelligence that can change a perception."

Colour can be used in therapy in many different ways. Specifically, Colour Mirrors explores how colour can reflect our internal world and what insights can be gained from this about the self, as well as life around us. This is done by connecting with the coloured essential oil bottles and essences.

The bottles can be held or intuitively placed on areas of the body, where you're able to connect with and absorb their energies. You can also rub droplets of the oil into your skin or bathe in the entire bottle's oil to fully absorb the frequencies. Essences can be sprayed into the air or onto the body. Another thing you can do is place a bottle beside your bed each night and allow yourself to absorb its energy whilst you sleep.

Upon connecting with a bottle, you may experience physical sensations or insights that occur. Each bottle has its own knowledge and information to share. It will share and help shift whatever is required specifically for each person. I find the shifts in awareness to sometimes be quite subtle. Other times they can be bold and dramatic—as if you're being reborn into a version of you that actually always existed within. That version of you was only dormant, waiting to be rediscovered.

How Colour Mirrors Is Beneficial

Colour Mirrors was able to create massive shifts and changes within me. It accelerated my personal growth in such a tremendous way. I was able to overcome significant blockages that had been outside of my awareness without me having to revisit the cause of the blockage.

My whole perspective on myself and life was transformed in a way where I never feel alone. I trust in the bigger picture as my life unfolds, moment by moment. I don't have to have it all figured out at once, or be in control of any future outcomes. Whatever happens, happens. I appreciate and value that experience for whatever it is. There's always something to be learnt or gained. Nothing happens in vain or is a waste.

I wholeheartedly believe that I never would've begun this book if it wasn't for this system. The colour copper solidified in me how to ground myself into taking fearless action, knowing that I'm always supported by Mother Earth and the universe itself.

Prior to my experience with the colour copper and its bottle's frequencies, I had a lot of ideas and plans, yet struggled to put them into consistent action. I would talk myself out of doing things with excuses or would get stuck daydreaming or phone scrolling, instead of just doing the thing!

Copper in the Colour Mirrors system really opened me up to me how alive Earth is with energy and that energy is beaming with love and support for us all. Gaia, is the name for our Earth, who sustains us with life and keeps us connected to her solid surface with gravity. I was able to overcome the feeling that I was an alien from another planet who didn't belong. I realised that I really am safe in all I do. I belong here and I'm connected to the Earth and all things of the Earth. It's my birthright to be here and enjoy life— or I wouldn't have been born nor would I have survived the near-death experiences I had.

That was a powerful realisation for me. For as long as I could remember, I had never felt like I belonged on the planet. It felt like I just didn't fit in here. I would sometimes joke about the moon being my home. I always had this innate sense of, *this isn't my home and why am I even here?*

It was like I had a diminished sense of motivation and drive to fully apply myself to life. Some days, I just didn't really care. What was the point in all of this wake, eat, work, play, sleep, repeat cycle? Yes, I did try with things and apply myself, but there were a lot of things I procrastinated on or just completely avoided. I also had this awesome habit of daydreaming and living in this fantasy world whilst allowing things to crash around me or deadlines to be missed. Checking emails and replying to messages? Give that one to two weeks on average to reply. Feeling as if I didn't belong was normal for me. At some stage, I accepted that I just didn't care enough to apply myself 100% anymore. People would say the word self-sabotage and I would think, what sabotage? Who cares, this is all meaningless and we will all die one day.

Integrating myself with the frequencies of the copper bottles helped me understand that there's no time except now. The present moment. The time is always now. I'm supposed to be here, taking action toward my future, or else I wouldn't be here with opportunities in front of me. I wouldn't be having the ideas to create in the first place. I felt revitalised and energised to take action.

It also helped me feel really connected with the Earth, feeling her unconditional love and support as a child of the planet. I'm safe, I'm nurtured. Even if the road gets tough or obstacles arise, I can ground into the Earth and my body. Then I remember how safe and supported I really am.

Being able to feel grounded, connected and safe within my own body may sound unusual to some. These feelings really help when experiencing dissociation symptoms due to trauma, which I was. I was able to get out of being stuck in my head (mental and emotional bodies). I now feel more confident in making capable decisions and steps for myself on the path forward. Not to mention feeling safe and supported even if something doesn't go to plan.

After these realisations, I took action and found the mentorship and support I would need to write this book (it had been an idea for a while but I had made the excuse to save it for later in life). The whole process just flowed. It was as if my new awareness had mirrored out into the world, creating a new reality for myself. I realise now that it's actually quite selfish to put it off. If I have the experience, knowledge, opportunity and ability to be able to write a book now, keeping it to myself isn't going to help or inspire anyone in the ways I have been. It takes a strong mindset. A wide variety of thoughts and feelings are stirred in the process of writing a book. Procrastination is also so easily done. I really do value the transformation I experienced upon working with the copper colours of this system.

Another experience I had with this system, was a shift that happened over time. Before Colour Mirrors, I had a subconscious belief it was weak to be soft and feminine. Prior to this system, I wasn't aware of this—I believed it was just my personality. I had been a tomboy when I was younger and became more feminine in appearance over time. However, I found it impossible to cry in front of others or to express authentic vulnerability. I also felt guilty for being still and not doing anything. I felt like I had to always be doing something, rather than sitting and just being. Thanks to my experiences with this system, I learned that I was rejecting my feminine side. I'm now able to embrace this side instead.

A quick crash course: we are comprised of both masculine and feminine energies, and some of us may feel more dominant in one or the other. This isn't biased to gender. Another part of being energetically balanced is having your feminine side balanced as well as your masculine side. This doesn't mean they need to be a 50/50 split. This means the feminine energy within you is balanced, which could be 70% of your energetic field, and the masculine energy within you is also balanced, and that makes up the remaining 30%.

From my experiences with connecting with the pinks, greens and rose golds of the Colour Mirrors, I now understand the beauty of being in touch with my soft, nurturing, feminine power. I'm able to express myself honestly with love and vulnerability. I also have no shame in asking for help or letting others know when I'm struggling. I don't feel like a victim of life and the trauma of my past. I understand that any time I feel or felt like a victim is an opportunity to listen to, love and nurture myself. I have become softer and gentler as I have realised I don't have to fight to prove or be anything. I'm loved and supported in my entirety. I just need to speak my truth with love and compassion, it doesn't have to be agreed on or accepted by anyone else. I also don't have to have all the answers figured out. I can just sit, and allow them to come to me instead.

Another story I will share is about bottle 19 in the system of "Buddhic Bliss". This bottle is comprised of pale magenta over gold. It relates to new beginnings and feeling pure bliss and love towards yourself, others and life itself. It's about embracing and expressing freedom and joy after challenging times. This bottle helps with letting go of guilt and shame, as well as recognising the divinity within yourself and all beings on the planet.

I decided to bathe in this bottle after feelings of guilt within myself kept arising. As uncovered initially in Dragon Magic Hypnotic sessions, I had this deep feeling inside that I was a bad person. I didn't deserve happiness and love in life. Remember previously I mentioned how healing isn't linear. Well, here I was revisiting this subconscious block. This time, these feelings had decided to come to the surface as I was stepping up to take on clients and share my wisdom with the world. I decided to bathe in bottle 19 to help me gain insight into what seemed to be an irrational fear of succeeding. I got into the water, closed my eyes and went into a meditative state.

I had visions of a magenta dragon flying me to a past life in ancient Rome. I was a guard/soldier. I had hurt and killed people on the basis of following orders in my job. I received guidance from the spiritual world to forgive myself because it all unfolded perfectly. Things had to happen the way they were supposed to so that in this lifetime I wouldn't be one to blindly follow orders or practice my spirituality for dark intentions. In this past life, I believed I was doing the right thing as the Roman army was asking the war god, Mars, for help in winning battles, as this was being granted.

Next, I was transported to a Japanese past life, before the Roman one. I was a lady in a hot spring. I was grieving and devastated. My husband had died in battle and we didn't have children. I wanted to avenge him and help fight in the war on his behalf but wasn't allowed to, being a woman. I felt like my life had no meaning and ended up drowning myself. I felt the sense that this is where my issues around co-dependency had mostly originated from. Living that life is also what inspired me to become a Roman soldier.

One of my spirit guides, who is a Japanese samurai, came forward and told me that they were my husband from that lifetime. Again, it was all perfect because it taught me there's no actual separation in life, even by death. Even across lifetimes, the spirit of my husband from a previous life had still been with me, supporting and guiding me, whether I realised it or not. I'm never alone. I'm so loved.

I believe I was taken on a journey through time to reveal everything truly is perfect and for me to forgive myself for past life choices. There's no need for guilt, everything has and will unfold as it's supposed to. We have all come here to experience, learn, and expand our conscious awareness in doing so. No single person has the power to stuff up the divine order of life. I realised I shouldn't be so hard on myself or take myself so seriously. It's okay to make what I may perceive to be a mistake. There's always a bigger picture. Sometimes we don't understand it until we look back in hindsight as to why something had to play out the way that it did.

Since bathing in this bottle, I feel carefree on the path forward. It's like a huge weight was lifted. I understand more profoundly just how connected and perfect everything is. Even if my human judgment deems it imperfect, there's a bigger picture. I have learnt to trust that things are unfolding exactly how they're supposed to, even when they don't make sense. Everything is happening for the greatest good of the world, not just for myself. Everything really is connected.

From this system, I had some major shifts happen that were truly life-changing. These shifts included embracing my authentic feminine power and self-assuredly taking on more responsibility by becoming a homeowner, as well as starting my wellness business and content creation, including writing this book.

Colour Mirrors really helped me turn my ideas and dreams into a reality. The shifts were so subtle as if the information from each colour had integrated with my own cell's information. I was able to overcome what was holding me back and take action with confidence—and be opened up on a deeper level to the magic of the universe and life whilst doing so.

So, you may be thinking, this all sounds silly. You're just playing with colours. What are we, in kindergarten?

The best way to figure out if it's real or not is to give it a go for yourself. It might come off as childish but I think a lot of the problems we have in life are linked to the tendency to take things too seriously. We get too stressed and find ourselves dreaming back to a simpler and more carefree time when we were children. Colour Mirrors really connects you with your inner child again. It opens you up to remember all the things you pushed aside or forgot when you were younger. It reminds you not to take life so seriously, to imagine, create and play your way through obstacles, like a child naturally does.

Another objection that comes up is that the bottles are too expensive.

I would recommend saving up if you're feeling really drawn to a particular bottle or set. It's worth investing in yourself. You're your biggest investment in life. Anything you invest into your own growth and development will pay off in the long run. I have found that the more I invest in myself, the more my finances naturally improve as an indirect result.

Another option is that you can have colour therapy sessions without purchasing any of the bottles yourself. This way you can still connect with and absorb the bottle's energetic frequencies in order to gain benefits. You do not have to own any of the bottles yourself to connect with them. Although bathing in them is considered the most potent way of integrating their benefits on a deep, cellular level.

You may also be questioning the validity of the whole science behind this chapter, or even this book.

I understand it can be a lot to wrap your head around these sorts of concepts, especially all at once. A lot of these things aren't common or mainstream knowledge, but that doesn't make it any less relevant or effective when it comes to health and wellness. As science and technology are advancing, a lot of previously unexplained phenomena, such as intuitive or psychic abilities, are becoming more understood. There's a whole unseen world out there and as humans, we only detect what our senses allow us to perceive. For instance, what about the spectrums of colour we can't detect that insects can?

Play with Colour

First, I would suggest experimenting with playing with different colours. See if you notice how different colours make you feel when you connect with them. Does blue make you feel at peace or sad? What feelings arise when you look at the colour red?

Linking back to the chakra balancing exercises, you may have noticed that balancing certain chakras was connected to particular colours and coloured crystals. Each chakra has a corresponding energetic frequency with a corresponding colour frequency. You can use the corresponding colour or any colour you feel drawn to, to help balance each chakra.

If you're feeling drawn to the Colour Mirrors system, I suggest visiting www.colourmirrors.com and clicking the subheading Message in a Bottle. There you can view the bottles and see what happens. Do you connect with one? What stands out? What repulses you? It's possible to connect with just images of the bottle alone.

Alternatively, *The Wisdom of the Colour Mirrors* book by Korani Connolly and Melissie Jolly has images of each bottle and goes into depth about their meanings.

Summary

Colour is another word for light. Light energy exists throughout the universe, including throughout you.

Colour Mirrors enables shifts and transformations to take place for people by using light frequencies to penetrate the body's cells. This enables healing to take place on a cellular level as each cell absorbs and combines with the new frequencies. This allows for a shift in awareness and perception that leads to a greater understanding and love for yourself, others and life in general.

All in all, Colour Mirrors has helped me have a brighter and lighter outlook. I have learnt to understand and appreciate all of the colours and shades we experience in life. My perspective truly was blown apart and transformed in ways I never could have imagined or planned—all whilst gently exploring and playing with colour! It's truly magical.

I do want to note that my realisations from connecting with the colour copper aren't specific to me. You too are also safe and supported on this planet. You too belong. You too have a purpose and a path you're currently taking. The time is also now for you. Whatever it is that you've been thinking about and putting off—it's safe and okay for you to take those steps, to make those changes. Tomorrow never comes, all we have is now. It doesn't have to be all figured out or all done at once, just focus on what's in front of you right now, and take that one step. Then focus on taking the next one, and the next. Before you know it, you're somehow flying!

This also goes for my realisations around stepping into my authentic feminine power and letting go of guilt and co-dependency. I'm no more special or supported than you. We are all loved and special and supported in our own ways. We all have a purpose. We all belong. We are all experiencing and learning in our own ways. We all have the ability to overcome whatever is holding us back or keeping us small.

Chapter Nine

Crystals and Metaphysics

"Energy cannot be created or destroyed; it can only be changed from one form to another."
– Albert Einstein

By now, you may be starting to gather that there's a whole unseen world out there. We often believed this as children, though we were later told this is all imagined and a made-up fantasy. A lot of us naturally disconnect and tune it out. The truth is that energy is everywhere. Everything in the universe is energy. We are constantly absorbing and emitting various frequencies of energy. My question is, would you rather be able to direct your energies to create a fulfilling life or just be absorbing and reacting to the energies around you?

Why Metaphysics?

I find metaphysical, including crystal, healing to be very valuable in improving overall health and well-being. Crystals draw in the natural energies of the earth and emit those frequencies into the environment around them. These frequencies can assist in bringing your body and its energetic field back into a state of harmony and balance. Having blockages or an imbalanced energetic field coincides with experiencing "disease" or "illness".

This isn't new knowledge either. Throughout history, crystals have been used for various purposes. Ancient civilisations considered crystals to be very valuable tools in daily life. Crystals were once worn on armour as protective stones for going into battle.

Metaphysics also suggests that the body can heal itself. Crystal and metaphysical knowledge can be used to help you tap into your body's ability to be able to regenerate and repair itself. Rather than acting as a band-aid treatment, metaphysical therapies help get to the root of the issue and work on clearing it so that it can be overcome.

Metaphysics also supports the use of natural medicines and remedies, which have fewer toxic chemicals and are better for the environment, as well as our overall health. This form of treatment also doesn't come with a cocktail of nasty new problems, called side effects, like pharmaceuticals tend to.

Did you know that in 2001, the pharmaceutical market was worth 390 billion USD? And that by the end of 2020, it was worth 1.27 trillion USD?

As a collective, we seem to be getting sicker and more ill, despite our technologies and knowledge. If pharmaceutical companies are making this much money, why aren't they investing it back into better remedies? Perhaps every patient cured is bad for business?

> *"It's important that public funds be spent in research directions that are pushing market frontiers rather than working in existing areas. This means funding research not only on drugs but also on areas like lifestyle changes, even if the profit potential is lower for Big Pharma as you cannot sell that change as you can sell a medicine."*
> **– Mariana Mazzucato**

> *"Any illness is a direct message to you that tells you how you have not been loving who you're, cherishing yourself in order to be who you're. This is the basis of all healing."*
> **– Barbara Brennan**

If you think this is nonsense, you can continue living life feeling disconnected, stressed out, anxious, sick and/or in pain. In a state of disease. Or you can try something new. What's the worst that can happen?

What Is Metaphysics?

Metaphysics is a branch of philosophy that studies the invisible world. That is everything beyond what we easily notice in the physical world, including the energies in our world. It's quite a wide topic. For the purposes of this book, I will be discussing how this relates to alternative therapies and the body's natural ability to heal itself.

Everything in the universe is energy, as quantum physics has proven. Energy is constantly moving or vibrating and contains information. So then, everything is vibration. Energies are noticed using our five senses, or they can be more difficult to pick up on. Energetic fields are groups of vibrations of energy that interact.

What vibrational frequency a certain energy field may have depends on the speed and intensity that the energy particles move at. Vibrational frequency is often the main difference between what is in the physical and what is in the unseen world. This is similar to the solids, liquids and gases school lesson we all had. Gases, for instance, vibrate at a different frequency to liquids and solids, which is why they take different forms.

Energetic fields constantly interact and are able to attract or repel each other based on their vibrational frequencies. Like energies tend to attract other like energies. Something that is said to have a higher vibration is believed to be more positive in nature. Whereas something considered to be low vibrational is said to be more dense or negative.

A higher frequency can repel a lower frequency. This means denser vibrating energies can be detoxed away with higher vibed ones. This is the basis of metaphysical or energy-based healing.

Lower frequencies can also repel higher frequencies, though. Alcohol and cigarettes are said to have a lower frequency. Hence they create a negative impact on our health as their frequency is absorbed by our own energy field.

This understanding is the basis of the Law of Attraction, made famous by Rhonda Byrne's book *The Secret*. You attract what you are. If you want to attract greater things in your life, you have to lift your own greatness to match first. Rhonda suggests doing this by practicing being more consciously aware using positive affirmations, thoughts and feelings.

Energy fields are everywhere throughout life and the universe. You alone generate a gigantic number of fields. These all interact with each other, as well as intermingle with the infinite amount being generated outside of you. Each individual cell and organ in your body radiates their own energetic fields.

Our planet Earth also creates energetic fields that interact with our own. Crystals, which are produced by the Earth, have their own energy frequencies. Their vibrations vary from crystal to crystal, though, they're usually considered high vibrational, as are many things naturally from the Earth, such as fresh water, plants, fruit and vegetables.

Energetic fields can be categorised as physical fields, meaning they can be easily measured, or as subtle fields, which are more difficult to detect, and likely invisible. Physical fields include sound and light/colour. Subtle fields can explain how qi energy exists, as well as psychic or supernatural experiences. Subtle fields are connected to physical fields.

Some of your body's subtle fields relate to the aura. These are fields connected by invisible energy channels, such as the chakras. The auric fields are a series of layers with different colours and vibrations. Each layer has a corresponding chakra which filters energy between your external and your internal worlds.

Chakras are able to transform qi energy into the physical energy the body uses to function. The physical, mental, emotional and spiritual bodies mentioned previously are also part of your auric fields. The following diagram shows the auric field layers.

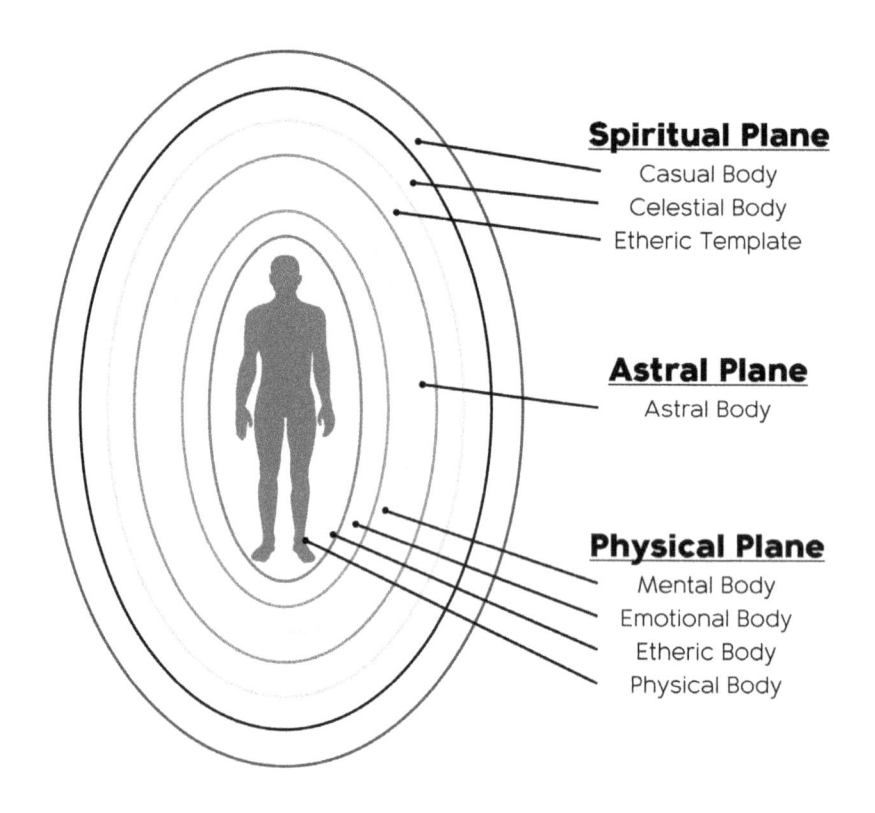

Spiritual Plane
Casual Body
Celestial Body
Etheric Template

Astral Plane
Astral Body

Physical Plane
Mental Body
Emotional Body
Etheric Body
Physical Body

How Is Metaphysical Knowledge Beneficial?

The basis of the alternative therapies I studied relies on metaphysical understandings of the body and the world.

Imagine we're like antennas for energy, bringing information in as well as sending energetic signals out into the world. When our energy field or auric layers have blockages from lower vibrational, denser energies, it causes the flow of energy to become stagnated. When the flow of energy within your energetic field is disrupted, your energy is imbalanced. This makes you more vulnerable to illness, injury or decreased well-being.

When the energy is flowing harmoniously, you're said to be balanced and in a state of optimal health and well-being. Many alternative therapies, such as the ones mentioned, work by clearing blocked and stagnated energetic fields. Usually, they're transformed into lighter and higher vibrational energies. As Einstein says, "Energy cannot be created or destroyed, only transformed."

Our physical, emotional, mental and spiritual bodies all have energetic fields, which can become blocked by lower vibrational energies. A blockage in one body may cause blockages in others. This is because all four bodies interact and influence each other to produce your overall health and well-being.

Metaphysical knowledge can assist us in understanding how to prevent or reduce the likelihood of poor health and well-being. It enables us to be more aware of what we are putting into our bodies, i.e. fast food (lower vibe) vs. healthier options (higher vibe). Also, activities such as spending time in nature or exercising, are said to help increase our vibration.

Emotions also have a vibrational frequency. Being in a state of gratitude, joy, love, peace and happiness is said to be higher vibrational than being in a state of despair, guilt, shame or anger. By working on clearing energetic blockages, we're able to improve our overall mood. This also works in the reverse. Practicing being grateful rather than complaining will help elevate your overall vibration and mood.

Remember the power of the mind and how our expectations can change our experience?

Thoughts also have energetic vibrations. Positive thoughts are said to be high and negative said to be lower. By focusing on shifting our thinking, we're able to shift our energetic vibration and overall well-being.

When blockages of energy occur in the auric layers or chakras, this information can transfer into the other energy bodies and manifest as disease. By using knowledge of energy and vibrations, these chakra blockages are able to be cleared, such as by using crystals, colour, Reiki, essential oils, sound or acupuncture. This allows energy to flow easily through your chakra system, which leads to better physical and mental health.

Alternative therapies have a tendency to focus on the root cause of an issue, rather than clearing the symptom of the problem. Energetic blockages are usually the root cause of why undesirable symptoms or feelings emerge.

These therapies also tend to view health and you as a whole being of various energies interacting with one another. They focus on the bigger picture, rather than separating you into your physical body or your mental health. You're a whole being after all.

Factors across all energetic fields tend to feed into and influence each other, resulting in what manifests into our reality. Whether that be feeling happy and healthy or feeling stressed and as if your health is falling apart.

This is how I was able to overcome chronic pain and stop medications. The medications I was prescribed were actually making me sicker. After years of being dependent on painkillers, I was getting some serious digestive issues as well as mental health side effects. Eventually, the painkillers weren't even helping the pain as my body grew tolerant. My quality of life seemed to be heading down a slippery slope.

With the power of the mind and Dragon Magic Hypnotic's help, I was able to clear energetic blocks in my mental body, i.e. subconscious, therefore overcoming the life of pain I was experiencing.

By clearing energetic blockages in my mental body, the energy was able to smoothly flow into my physical body.

Smoothly flowing energy meant smooth exchanges of information between my body's various energy fields. This enabled my mind to easily work with my body's cells and organs to heal itself! I had significantly reduced pain and grew stronger and healthier over time. I was able to function again without medications.

Not only is metaphysical knowledge beneficial for our health, but it's also wonderful for reconnecting us back to the planet and our natural roots. I keep mentioning the importance of our planet and the environment because, without our Earth, we wouldn't have life.

Everything in life is so connected and affects each other. I think it's important we take care of the Earth and adopt the natural resources it provides. They're energetically really healthy for us compared to man-made alternatives which tend to create more blockages. Producing man-made alternatives is also harmful to the planet due to the toxic and chemical by-products. Perhaps energy doesn't lie.

Not to mention, our ancestors and ancient civilisations once relied on the planet's natural medicines for health and well-being. Plant medicines and crystals were widely adopted by many cultures. The higher vibrations of plants and crystals are able to repel lower vibrations from the body. Detox symptoms, such as a cold or diarrhea, may arise as they are expelled as toxins. It's normal to experience them as you're flushing out lower vibrational energies that were once stored within you. This is similar to the side effects that arise when beginning a healthy detox diet.

I find crystals in particular to be really powerful tools for improving health and well-being. Different crystals have different energies which have varying benefits depending on the stone. They draw on the natural vibrations of the Earth and store this energetic information within them. This information can be absorbed by your own energy field and have an influence on you.

As each crystal has different energetic purposes, I really like using them as tools to amplify the work I do with clients, as well as to support my own well-being.

Black stones, such as obsidian or black tourmaline, are very effective as protective stones. They're able to absorb lower vibed energies so that you don't. I like to keep black crystals on my desk, in between myself and my laptop, to help protect me against harmful radiation waves.

Rose quartz emits frequencies of pure love and calm. It's great for reducing anxiety and sadness. I enjoy meditating with rose quartz in the centre of my chest, where the heart chakra is. I find the energies to be so calming and they help fill me with feelings of bliss, especially after experiencing heartbreak.

Selenite is amazing for cleansing and purifying low vibe energies, which may have become stuck or stagnated. I like to keep selenite in my bedroom so it can cleanse the energy in my room and myself whilst I sleep. Placing other crystals against selenite will also cleanse those crystals of any lower vibrations they may have absorbed.

Crystals and Metaphysics

Crystals do need regular cleansing and charging to work at an optimal level, as they can become blocked with low vibrational energies as we can. Perhaps you haven't felt the magic of crystal energy because the crystal's you've interacted with haven't been cleansed and charged!

You may be wondering why isn't this knowledge widely accepted by science or the medical world if it's real. Wouldn't it be everywhere and commonly understood?

Our past ancestors and civilisations throughout history have used this knowledge to help themselves. This wisdom seems to have been lost or forgotten, yet is being rediscovered in recent times. I find this exciting because maybe we can combine the knowledge of the medical world with metaphysical understandings. Perhaps the two can amplify one another in assisting our overall well-being.

I'll also put forth that the pharmaceutical industry seems to be driven largely by profits. This industry may not be motivated to adopt this knowledge into their treatments as every patient cured is a customer lost. In the world we live in, lots of things are sold to us for money.

You might also be thinking that metaphysics isn't real.

Quantum physics, a newer branch of physics, has emerged in recent times. This field is making discoveries that support these concepts around energy and how it works. I think it's the bridge that explains how these alternate therapies actually work. It's possible to have a PhD in quantum physics, it's real.

You still may be thinking this is delusional and made up.

That's okay, you don't have to adopt my perspective. I'm impressed you've made it this far into the book, though. Perhaps some part of you is open to the possibility of energy healing being beneficial.

Tap into the Mystical World

If you didn't do it in the Reiki chapter, practice feeling energies!

If you can feel the differences in energies despite not being able to see them, it will help you understand their existence.

It's like the air. We might not be able to see the air, but we can feel it and we know it's real from that. You could also try to notice differences in energies in rooms or buildings. Does the energy in a room feel different after an argument or heated situation has happened?

Another step you could take is to go out and buy a crystal that you're drawn to and see what happens. See if you can notice any differences when you hold or tune into it. I find meditating with crystals beneficial as I receive helpful insights from them. They really are lovely, supportive companions. Don't forget to cleanse and charge them. This can be done in many ways. One way you can cleanse them is by using incense or sage smoke. A way they can be charged is under the full moon's light or in the sunshine.

Finally, you could practice seeing subtle energy fields such as auras. I find it easier to try to see your own aura first, especially against a white background in dim lighting. Squint your eyes so that they are just open and see if you can notice any differences around your body or another form. Try not to focus too hard with your vision. You may, at first, be able to distinguish subtle layers of energy or colours surrounding you or the form you're observing.

Summary

Everything in the universe is energy. Energetic fields exist everywhere and constantly interact with and impact one another.

Energetic frequencies can be high or low vibration. Higher vibrations are linked to higher states of health and well-being. Lower vibrations are linked to states of disease or illness as they can create blockages in your energetic bodies or fields. Your body has the ability to heal itself naturally when running optimally, i.e. these blockages are cleared.

Alternative therapies and natural medicines are effective because they help to remove these blockages and raise the vibration of your energetic field. Crystals are high-vibrational tools from the Earth which can be used to help enhance your health and well-being.

Chapter Ten

Go Within

"Meditation is not about stopping thoughts, but recognizing that we are more than our thoughts and our feelings."
– Arianna Huffington

All the answers that you need are within you. There's a whole world inside of you to explore. The state of that internal world is often re-experienced in the world outside of us.

Why Meditation?

Firstly, it's literally rest for the brain.

When you're sleeping, your brain is actually super active. It's busy processing, organising and filing everything away from the previous day. It's also busy dreaming. So, when you sleep, your brain isn't actually resting all that much. Although sleep is still an important process for your brain's health, meditation is like an actual break or rest for it.

Meditation also helps connect you with your own intuition or inner voice. Your inner guidance is a good compass to follow in life. There's a lot of wisdom in intuitive knowledge. How many times have we gone against our gut feeling only to realise we were right all along?

Meditating assists with being less reactive. You come to understand that you're not your thoughts in your mind. You're merely the observer of these thoughts. Meditating is simply practicing the observation of your thoughts without attaching to them as being a part of you and true.

It also helps with focusing on the present moment rather than mentally being stuck in the past or anxious about the future. A lot of mental unrest occurs when we're dwelling on the past or worried about the future. Meditation helps with letting go of these two and focusing on what is happening currently. For these reasons, meditation is fantastic for reducing stress and supporting feelings of inner peace.

Did you know that meditation changes the structure of your brain by increasing its amount of grey matter? All of the information processing your brain does happens in the grey matter areas. If you have more grey matter, your brain is more effective at how it processes and interprets the information it receives.

"If you see the world in black and white, you're missing important grey matter."
— **Jack Fyock**

"I meditate so that my mind cannot complicate my life."
— **Sri Chinmoy**

If you don't meditate, you can stay living life with racing thoughts, and then reacting to those thoughts and your environment, mindlessly. Or you can take charge of your own inner world and connect with a greater sense of peace.

Getting a grip on your inner world will allow your daily life to flow more easily. There always will be obstacles. Healing or overcoming trauma isn't about eliminating obstacles. Healing is about changing our perspective and how we respond to whatever obstacles emerge.

What Is Meditation?

Meditation is exercise for your brain. It involves entering a state of stillness, usually seated or laying down with your eyes closed. It's a state of focusing on something whilst also observing what passes through the mind. I usually focus on my breath or the centre point between my eyebrows.

In this state of observing, you practice paying attention to your thoughts without attaching any meaning to them. Meditating is about learning to observe the thoughts and feelings that arise within you, without judging or labelling them. It's the art of simply noticing your thoughts drift in and out of your mind, without holding onto or getting stuck in any thought patterns.

There are many different ways of meditating, such as mindfulness or breathwork. I like to practice mindfulness meditation which focuses on becoming present in the moment. Mindfulness is being aware of yourself and what you're experiencing in the current moment, without being reactive or judgmental. It's a state of observation.

Mindfulness meditation can be practiced at all times, you just have to simply tune into your breath and focus on what's in front of you without judging something as good or bad. Just noticing it with all its detail for what it is.

In mindfulness meditation, I like to focus on my breath as I find it helps me detach from the thoughts travelling through my mind. I like to get comfortable and close my eyes. I slow my breathing and focus on each in and out breath. I observe what sensations are occurring in my body, as well as what my senses are picking up on in the world around me.

I focus on my breath whilst doing this and allow my thoughts to drift in and out of my mind. If a judgmental thought comes into my mind, I try not to react to it with more judgment of whether it's good or bad. I tend to think *that was interesting* as I let it leave my awareness, and the next thought enters. The aim is to try to neutralise your responses to your thoughts as much as possible.

I want to note that it's commonly misunderstood that the goal of meditation is to empty your mind. This is untrue! The goal of meditating is to slow the thinking process down and let go of judgmental or reactive thoughts that lead to negative feelings or overreactions. It's about practicing expanding your awareness so you learn to become the observer of your thoughts, rather than identify as being a part of your thoughts.

When you learn to view things in life as neutral, rather than good or bad, a greater sense of inner peace is established. Challenges and obstacles won't disappear, however, we become better at handling them.

I also find guided meditations really helpful. Especially, if you're struggling with meditating on your own. It helps to have a guided track or even just some nice relaxing music if you're struggling to unwind.

How Is Meditation Beneficial?

Meditation is beneficial as it's able to help change the structure of your brain, particularly in increasing grey matter. Having more grey matter means your brain has a stronger ability to process all information. This means you become more equipped at handling stressful situations, being more present in the current moment, and gaining better concentration and clarity.

An analysis of 18 studies[5] demonstrated that meditation as a therapy was able to improve symptoms of depression in people, compared to those who didn't receive any meditation treatment.

Meditating regularly helps you connect with your inner world on a deeper level. By learning to observe and slow our thoughts, we're more clearly able to notice guidance from our heart and gut instincts.

Cells similar to brain neurons have been found within the heart as well as the digestive system. This explains the phenomena of our gut instincts and how we can make decisions led by the heart and not the mind.

I have found learning to balance my brain mind, heart mind and gut mind to be super beneficial when navigating through life. Our inner knowing has so much wisdom to share with us. It really is limitless. Sometimes the brain overcomplicates things or keeps us in a state of comfort which becomes counterproductive.

Personally, I first started meditating when I was still at university completing my psychology degree. It really helped improve my productivity so I could get through assignment and exam stress, whilst juggling a part-time job.

I would be so mentally exhausted from my days. I would do a 10- to 20-minute meditation in my car around that "3:30-itis time" when the mental fog kicked in. I found this would re-energise and reset me as if I had taken a refreshing nap (not one of those ones where you wake up feeling more tired after). It was like having a coffee!

After my uni days, I fell out of the habit and didn't feel as aligned and in flow as I had prior. I found myself more reactive to stressors again, getting stuck in catastrophic thinking patterns about how shit everything was. Everything really did turn to shit after my uni degree—what with the domestic violence and the car accident!

It wasn't until after those two traumas, back-to-back, that I began practicing meditation again. I had become a mess and my mind was spiralling. Although I needed additional help with Dragon Magic Hypnotic, meditating in my own time also helped me get back into a state of inner harmony. I found it helped me a lot with panic attacks.

Practicing meditating enabled me to slow the whole trigger-thought and emotion-react response. I was able to slow the whole process down by tuning into my breath. I got better at noticing when I was being triggered so I became less reactive. I learnt to follow my breath so that I could stop and assess, "Am I actually in danger? No? Okay, this is just a trigger, I'm safe. How can I defuse this so I don't panic?"

Usually, the solution involved removing myself from the environment so that I could reset and calm down before I caused complete chaos around me. Mindlessly causing complete chaos around me due to triggers from trauma was once a specialty of mine. Now it's a specialty of mine to be able to mindfully observe my internal state and respond accordingly.

You may be thinking that you suck at meditating because you just fall asleep.

Perhaps you needed that bit of sleep at the time. Perhaps you just went into a deep trance-like state that felt like sleep. If you're listening to guided meditations when you fall asleep, your subconscious mind is still listening and benefiting. You may not have been consciously aware, but your subconscious is always listening.

You could always set a timer or alarm at the beginning of a meditation so that if you do nod off, you will be woken again. It's okay to fall asleep, but the aim is to enter a focused, relaxed state. Learning to focus whilst relaxing will come as you practice meditating.

You may also think that you suck at meditating.

That's okay, it takes practice. Start small. It's like any skill. Imagine it as similar to building muscle at the gym. You're not going to be perfectly strong at lifting weights straightaway. I remember when

I first started, I could only meditate for like a minute, and then that was it. I just built my way up from one minute to two and so on. It gets easier.

You may have also experienced getting stuck meditating on racing thoughts which spiral and worsen your mood.

A strategy I would recommend is to try to imagine your thoughts moving through your mind as clouds. Just relax and watch them float by. Don't judge them as good or bad clouds. Notice them as they are, and let them drift away.

Another visualisation people like to use is that same process but imagining thoughts as leaves on a river stream, or balloons floating up into the sky. It's honestly up to you.

There's no right or wrong way of meditating. The main point is to be spending time out of your day in stillness, where you draw your attention to observing your internal world instead of everything that is happening around you.

If mindfulness or guided meditations really aren't your thing. I would highly recommend checking out breathwork as it's a more active form of meditation that some people prefer as it keeps them more focused on their breath than their thoughts.

Being Mindful

Firstly, I would recommend having a go at doing a guided meditation, even if it's just five to 10 minutes in your morning. I like to do it first thing as it sets you up well for the day. Try it and see if there's a difference in how your day plays out.

If you have trouble falling asleep, I would recommend putting on a guided meditation before you go to bed. This will help slow your thoughts and get your brain into a state for you to more easily fall asleep. There are plenty of amazing free guided meditation tracks on YouTube.

A simple meditation exercise I like to do with myself is to sit with my feet planted on the floor. I imagine a ball of pure, loving, golden light coming down from the sky above and entering the top of my head. I visualise it travelling down my body and into my heart. I then spend time connecting with this healing light and really feel its gentle, healing energy. Try it yourself and see if you notice any colours, sensations or visions coming through.

I'd also recommend doing small mindfulness exercises, such as when you're driving your car. See if you can practice observing your experiences and thoughts in the present moment without judgment.

When I'm driving my car, I like to tune into my breathing and just observe the traffic around me as I drive along. The trick is to practice not reacting to other drivers by thinking they're idiots or the usual road rage. Instead, focus on observing what they're doing without labelling them as a good or bad driver.

Notice the colours, shapes and speeds of the cars and practice letting go of labels which evoke emotional responses from you. What is the weather and scenery like? Notice how you feel inside of yourself when you shift your perspective from judgment to observation.

I highly suggest practicing observing your thoughts, without identifying with them as if they are you. If a thought enters your mind that is quite harsh, try not to react to it or judge yourself as terrible for thinking that.

For example, normally you might react to that thought with, *that's horrible as if I thought that,* and let that thought pattern take you on a ride of judgment and more negative thoughts.

Instead, practice thinking, *wow, that was interesting* and letting it fade as quickly as it appeared in your mind. It's normal for us to have some questionable thoughts enter our minds. What determines our character is how we respond to those initial thoughts, not the thoughts themselves.

Summary

Meditation is like exercise and a nap for your mind. It helps slow down thinking and promotes greater feelings of resilience when it comes to stress and depression.

Meditation tunes you into your internal world so that you can be less reactive toward what happens in your environment.

Meditation helps us strengthen the observation of thoughts without judgment. You're not your thoughts. You're the observer. You don't have to listen to or react to everything that you think.

Your being is so much more than that voice in your head. You have a mind in your heart and a voice in your gut too. Mindfulness and meditative practices strengthen our connection with these minds.

Being tuned into your inner world and inner wisdom will improve your quality of life compared to if you're just attaching to your thoughts all day.

Chapter Eleven

Physical Vessel

"Our bodies are our gardens – our wills are our gardeners."
– William Shakespeare

As our inner world is important, so is what connects our inner world to the outer world…our physical body.

Why Take Care of Your Physical Health?

I know you've perhaps heard it abundantly before. Your body is your temple!

I definitely learned this when recovering from the car accident and surgeries. If you don't have your health, you really don't have much else. Every other activity you love usually requires a certain level of health to participate.

Being stuck in a bed or hospital due to poor health really is an eye-opener. You can't go to work and earn income. You can't visit your loved ones. You can't shower without help. You start to realise how dependent everything else is on your body's health. For this reason, I like to say that your health is your wealth. Prevention is key. I would recommend prioritising your physical health as best you can.

Taking care of your physical body or vessel is also a form of self-love and self-care. You live inside of your body from the day you're born until the day you die. You're much more than the physical vessel you exist within—you are a life force with a soul. Your body is the home where your essence is stored whilst you inhabit the planet during this lifetime. It's still important and a part of your being! Taking care of your health and body is a form of self-respect and a way to honour yourself.

Looking after your physical health will also help increase your vibration. Memories and emotions are stored in the cells of tissues within the body. This is called cellular memory and explains the phenomena where people have reported feeling like parts of their personality have changed after undergoing organ transplant surgery. Cellular memories stored in the organ from a donor can get transferred into the body of the receiver.

Information from past experiences or even past lives is encoded into our cell's DNA. Thus, trauma and its effects are also stored in your body's cells. Remember negative emotions are considered to be lower in vibration. This means their denser energies can remain stagnated and blocked within your body's cells. Taking care of your body's health will help you detox toxins and stagnated energies faster than not. On a side note, Reiki works by helping to purify cellular memories from the body's cells and energy field.

Looking after your physical health also helps with being more grounded in your body, as well as the Earth itself. I have found this to be exceptionally important when overcoming the effects of trauma on the body, such as dissociation or derealisation. Being grounded leads to greater feelings of safety and security in life. This usually indicates your root chakra is balanced.

Finally, taking care of your physical body helps you with feeling more confident as you become physically fit and healthier. Seeing yourself gain progress by eating reasonably well and exercising regularly will boost your confidence in smashing goals in other areas of life. When you feel and look great, your well-being is automatically enhanced.

A relationship exists between your mind and body. Taking care of your physical health has significant positive impacts on your emotional and mental health. Better emotional and mental health also has positive impacts on your physical health.

> *"After trauma the world is experienced with a different nervous system. The survivor's energy now becomes focused on suppressing inner chaos, at the expense of spontaneous involvement in their lives. These attempts to maintain control over unbearable physiological reactions can result in a whole range of physical symptoms, including fibromyalgia, chronic fatigue, and other autoimmune diseases. This explains why it's critical for trauma treatment to engage the entire organism, body, mind, and brain."*
> **– Bessel A. van der Kolk**

"To keep the body in good health is a duty...otherwise we shall not be able to keep the mind strong and clear."
– Buddha

If your body becomes your enemy because you're abusing or neglecting it, it will continue down that spiral until it eventually suffers illness or disease. By this point, your mental, emotional and/or spiritual health would have likely spiralled downwards also. Everything is connected and operates holistically.

Do you want to be at war with your body or do you want to work alongside it?

Your body works so hard to keep itself alive and functioning as optimally as it can.

Wouldn't you rather work towards that same goal?

It seems counter-productive to even create unnecessary harm and risks for your body!

What Is Your Physical Body?

Well, if you think about it. Our body is the sacred vessel we live inside of that requires certain needs to be met for our survival. On an energetic level, our physical body consists of universal matter that vibrates slowly enough that it can be easily noticed by our five senses.

Chakras act as filters between the external world and our internal world, including our physical body. When we take care of our physical health, such as through diet and exercise, our chakras are going to be more balanced. This means that energy is more likely to flow easily between your energetic bodies, and energy fields in your environment.

When a person experiences trauma or stress, the effects can be felt in not only their mind but also within their physical body. Your body stores tension and stress within your cell's memory. If not released, this tension can build up until a breaking point is reached. Breaking points can come in the form of chronic illness, mental breakdowns and burnout.

How Is Taking Care of Your Physical Health Beneficial?

In order to better understand this concept, I will explain the stress response. When a person experiences or perceives a threat or danger, their fight or flight response is activated. This response can also include freezing in fear.

In the wild, this response is very advantageous as it tells us how to respond if we cross paths with a tiger. In today's society, not only traumatic events but also everyday stressors can trigger a person's fight or flight response.

Repetitively being in this state can lead to various consequences and health detriments. This is referred to as being stuck in survival mode. One reason for this is cortisol, the stress hormone, is released by the adrenal glands. At healthy levels, cortisol is important for forming memories and regulating metabolism and blood sugar levels. It also supports a reduction in inflammation.

However, in large, frequent quantities, cortisol can be fairly damaging to our overall health. Prolonged body cortisol levels can bring about symptoms such as severe burnout, irritability, concentration issues, weight gain, muscle weakness, acne and high blood pressure.

Being stuck in survival mode distracts you from focusing on solutions and what will help you thrive in life. This is because you're often hypervigilant about imminent danger and preoccupied with meeting your basic survival needs. These include feeling safe or financially secure.

If most of your energy is being expended on surviving, then of course you will feel too drained and unwell to live a happier, calmer life. This is why taking care of your physical health is important. It's beneficial to keep the state of your physical body in harmony so that you can more easily balance your mental, emotional and spiritual bodies. Having high cortisol levels disrupts this harmony.

Remember, the root or base chakra is connected with your feelings of security and survival needs. By taking care of your physical body, it will also help balance this chakra so that energy more freely flows as your vibration is elevated. The root chakra also relates to feeling grounded within your physical body.

What Is Grounding and How Does it Help?

Grounding is a technique which helps keep you in the present moment, rather than the thoughts in your mind or mental body. You can ground yourself by going on walks in nature or doing any exercise—including yoga, practicing mindfulness, and dancing. Using your body for creative expression, such as painting or creating art is also another way.

Mainly, I find walking barefoot with my feet on the ground like the grass, dirt or sand at the beach really fantastic. There are so many receptors in the soles of your feet that interact with the Earth energetically and connect us with it. We are all electromagnetic and it helps connect our field with the Earth's energetic fields. This supports a greater sense of belonging in the world.

The goal for grounding is to take part in an activity that connects you to your body and is happening in the present moment. Often, when we are stressed or have experienced trauma, we can feel detached or disconnected. One common by-product is dissociation, which is feeling disconnected from your sense of self and or surroundings.

In my experience, grounding is superb in solving issues around having a mind-body imbalance or disconnect. Sometimes we can get stuck in our mental body. This isn't rare for society. I think due to stress, a lot of us naturally find ourselves stuck in our thinking states, rather than actually doing. We can become too attached to our thoughts. This causes us to get "stuck in our heads" by getting trapped in analysis paralysis. We over-analyse rather than take action steps. A lot of great ideas come, but what steps are we actually taking?

When you feel grounded in your body and the Earth, you enhance a sense of connectedness to yourself and the planet. This helps with feeling less focused on issues in your life, as well as with living in the now moment. Being grounded in the here and now, rather than mental stressors, aids in decreasing your body's cortisol levels. When we experience anxiety, we are often too fixated on the future. When experiencing a depressive state, we are often too fixated on the past. Being engrossed in the current moment is enormously helpful—as we realise all we really have is this exact moment, now. That is all we need to focus on. The rest can slip away until it needs your attention.

Focusing on the present moment and making changes where we can today is how we can create a better future for ourselves. Stress and anxiety tend to hold us back from making changes or moving forwards with our goals. Being too stuck in the past can also hold us back from succeeding in future goals. We all have the power to change, as we all have the power of the current moment. *The Power of Now* by Eckhart Tolle is an excellent book which goes into further detail on this concept.

In my own personal life, after I had left the abusive relationship, I rediscovered my passion for art. This initially got me grounded. I was so fixated on the anxious thoughts in my head and felt disconnected from myself and the people around me. I quickly realised that the only place I felt safe and okay was when I was creating paintings.

Being creative took me away from the feelings of guilt and shame I had about the past. It also distracted me from the sheer terror and panic about what could happen in the future. I could get completely lost in the moment, even if it were only for an hour or two. It was giving my mind a rest from the racing, petrified thoughts that I had been existing in for too long.

When I'm painting, the mental and emotional stuff that exists within is able to find an outlet where it can be expressed. Again, as Einstein says, "Energy cannot be created nor destroyed, only transformed!"

Creative expression helps to transform denser energies trapped inside from trauma into something beautiful or meaningful. It's a wonderful way for your soul to express itself all whilst connecting you back in with your body and the world. I still paint today and the following are images of what I have created.

Physical Vessel

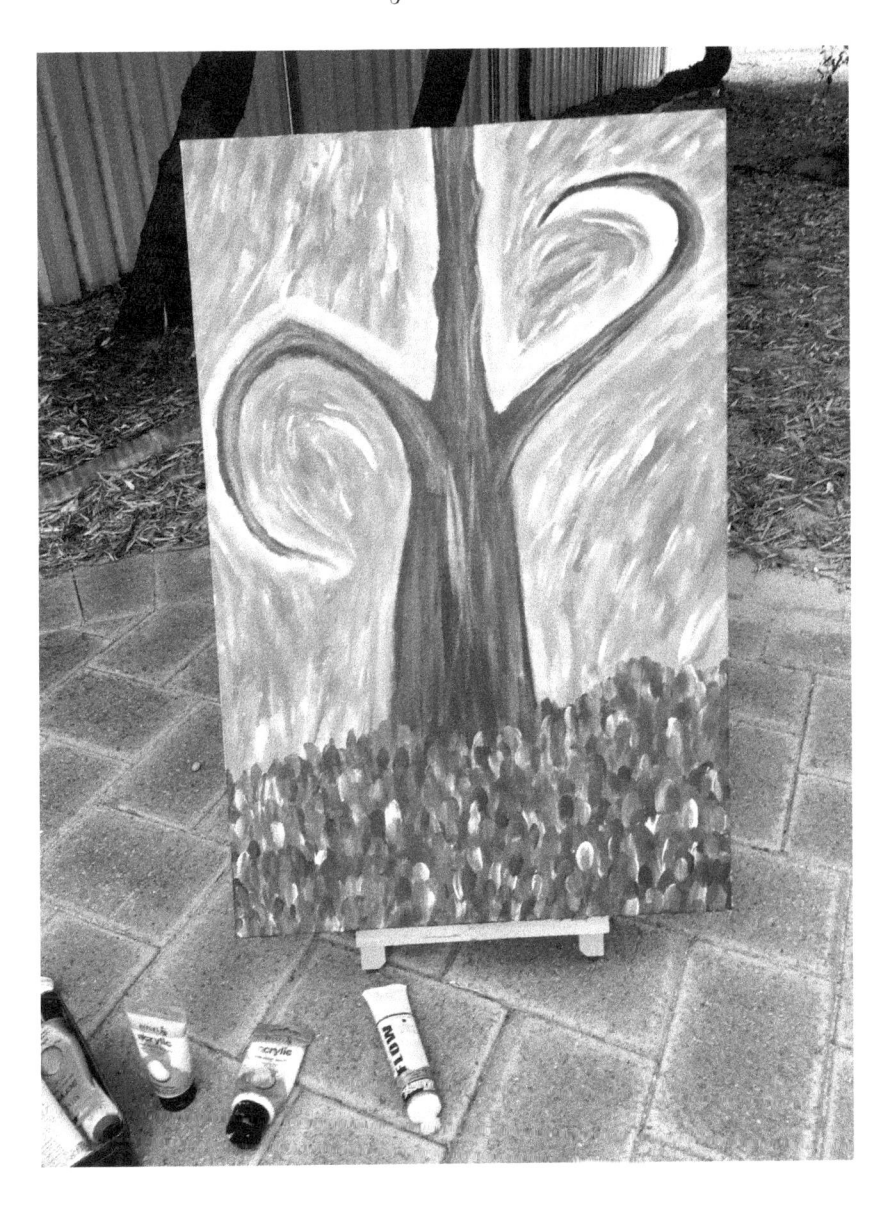

Having the car accident taught me an all-new relationship with my actual body. I had been reasonably fit throughout my life. After the pain and fatigue brought on by injuries, my body became my enemy. I had felt stuck and hopeless. It was like I was trapped inside a body which hurt and held me back.

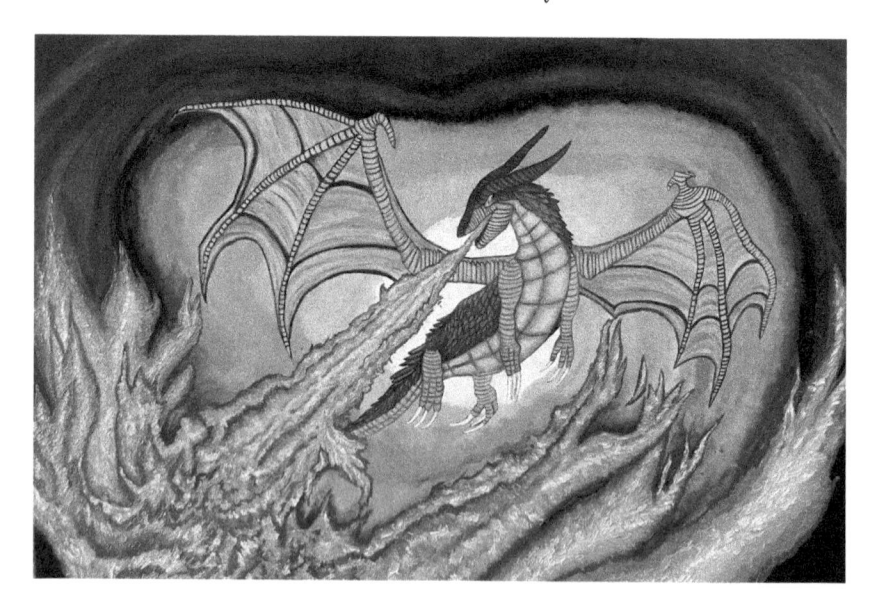

This fed into my mental and emotional health. That then caused more stress and depression (I was still recovering from the domestic violence trauma). The pain existing in my mental and emotional bodies then fed back into my physical body, worsening the physical pain I was suffering.

It was this never-ending loop because things weren't balanced. Instead of creating harmony between my energy bodies, I was creating conflict and it just kept accelerating.

You might be thinking that this is all boring. I want to have fun and put what I want into my body. Life is too short. I don't want a healthy lifestyle.

My response to that is that's 100% okay! You don't have to do it. However, taking care of your physical body's health is a form of self-care that I believe we should all honour. Our health is our wealth. You only need to do what you feel will help you or feel motivated or drawn towards doing. You don't have to force

Physical Vessel

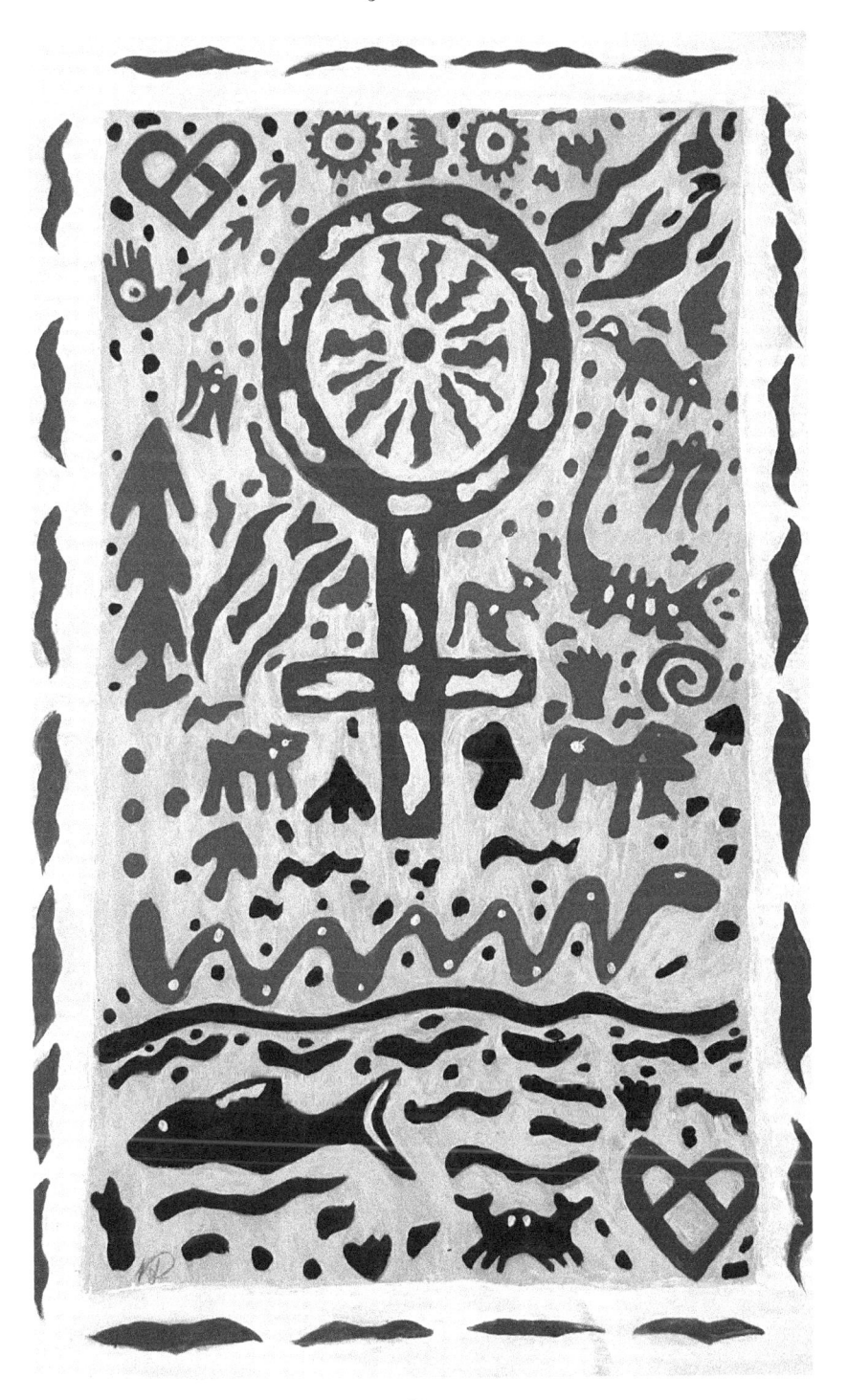

yourself to do anything based on my recommendations. Balance and moderation are key. You don't have to give something up forever if you don't want to. That's okay. You don't have to deprive yourself or make yourself miserable if that's what it's going to do. However, that feeling of deprivation may only be a short-term discomfort whilst you adjust to a newer, healthier way of being. At the end of the day, you know what's best for you. I'm only sharing what made a huge difference in my life.

You might be thinking that grounding sounds like a load of garbage.

Well, as someone who used to get very dissociated and disconnected from my body, after trauma, I've found grounding really, really powerful and helpful. I used to get stuck in a lot of frozen states where I would be fixated on the overthinking that was happening in my head. I was always distracted and never fully present. Grounding sure helped me go from fearful thinking, to confidently actually doing.

Another objection you may have is, if diet and exercise are so beneficial, why do we have medications?

I will make it clear that I'm not against medications. I think they serve their purpose but also there are alternative ways to help which seem to get to the root of the problem, rather than band-aid it. I will ask though, how many people do you actually know that have a really good diet and exercise? Are they healthy or are they sick all the time?

I know in my case, doing the energetic healing work really helped fix the side effects that painkillers, especially, gave me. I had been on painkillers for years. I was hardly able to eat. For a while, I thought I had stomach ulcers that just weren't clearing up, even with medicine. One day I went and got a scan done and it was found I had parasites throughout my intestines. My digestive system's health had been weakened from my painkiller use. I used natural remedies and powders to flush them out. Within two weeks, I went from struggling to finish one piece of toast to being able to eat a big breakfast, plus three or four more meals throughout the day.

I think it's important that we all treat our gut health for parasites at least once a year. We are going to naturally pick them up but they can wreak so much havoc on you and cause so much illness. Parasites can even affect your thinking and emotions without you even realising. For myself, they were mostly affecting my energy levels and digestion. So honestly, if you take one thing from this book, it's please heal your gut. Your gut is linked to your mind's health.

How to Care for Your Physical Health

For my part, I found a huge aspect of being in pain was linked to getting the right nutrition.

It's drilled into us continually from childhood…eat your vegetables! Having a good diet really does help with your body's ability to function optimally and repair itself. It's that simple. If you don't have the right fuel, how will things run properly?

Lacking certain vitamins and minerals can send your body into disharmony, disease or illness. I found taking magnesium and zinc supplements particularly helped with pain and stress levels.

Limiting your intake of processed food and drinks, cigarettes and drugs will have tremendous positive impacts. I have found that even limiting just soft drinks at the beginning made a hugely positive impact, particularly for my gut health.

Another way to care for your health is to get moving—exercise or walk daily. If you go walking, try to spend some of it barefoot on the grass, dirt or beach sand.

Get creating! It doesn't have to be art, although everyone has the ability to paint, draw and be an artist. It's about the expression of your inner world, more than the perceived quality of the work. Playing an instrument, cooking, interior decorating, gardening and dancing are other ways that you could be creative. Perhaps your creativity is through problem solving such as in mathematics? Explore your options and see what you enjoy the most.

Summary

It's important to take care of your physical health and body.

The moment my physical body was damaged, it was almost like I lost everything. I realised how much I had taken it for granted. How now all my other once huge problems seemed so small. I struggled to even just spend time with friends. I couldn't go socialise because I'd be in so much pain. I'd be exhausted. My physical health fed into every other area of life. I wasn't able to work and make money. I was spending a lot of money on medications and all these different doctors. I really felt trapped in a body that was my own worst enemy.

Taking care of my body and getting grounded really helped me break this cycle. I was able to thrive rather than survive.

Chapter Twelve

No Mistakes

"You always meet failure on your way to success."
– Mickey Rooney

We all make mistakes. Even the most successful people have failed their way to the top.

I think one of the biggest things in life that we face is the fear of making a blunder. Our education system sets us up where we are almost taught that making an error is wrong. We learn to associate mistakes with being bad and getting it right as correct. This is because we're rewarded when we're right. However, errors are an essential part of learning. We learn more from our faults than we do from being right.

I think it's important to understand there's no such thing as mistakes because it takes the pressure off of life in general. The meaning of life is to experience, which we are always doing without even trying. From the moment we are born until death, we're continuously going through life in some shape or form.

Our experiences, good and bad, are what mould us into the unique and special individuals that we are. When you understand that the meaning of life is simply to have experiences from the lows to the highs, then the pressure lifts off of making a mistake. Mistakes become just an experience that adds to the meaning of your life, your story. It's not right or wrong. It's neutral. There becomes less weight on making an error, therefore, less stress to get everything perfect. Life becomes more joyful, carefree and fun—like when you were a kid!

Throughout our lifespans, we're always learning. We're simultaneously students and teachers of life until our very last moment. There's always a different way of looking at something. There's always something to be learnt. We can't be expected to be perfect at everything.

Even if we fail or do wrong—we have gained insight. We have learnt something that will be encoded into our cellular memory. Our consciousness is further expanded. When our consciousness increases, we grow. The more we develop our awareness, the more humanity collectively evolves as a species.

However, God or source energy, the all-loving essence in everything, puts no pressure or rush on us to evolve. Time on Earth is different from how time functions in the cosmos. As everything is energetic vibration, everything is linked. We're all connected to this godly essence and everything around us is connected to it. As we progress, God also grows as this spirit learns through us.

Our mistakes help the higher realms understand and learn too, as they cannot live as humans.

We don't need to hurry ourselves or our healing. In fact, too much pressure creates disharmony instead of relaxingly flowing through life, viewing experiences as neutral. You can simply just look out at nature to remind you of this. Nature doesn't know mistakes. It just does what it does each day. Nature is not in a hurry either.

The only person who thinks they're in a rush or that they have to get it all right is you. Yeah, other people might pressure you. But that's external. You don't have to listen to them. You can shut that out. It's just distracting noise. You can detach.

So as long as we're experiencing, which we always are, then we are where we're supposed to be. It really is that simple. Don't let fear of failure hold you back. Normalise being okay with being unsuccessful—the most successful people are okay with this. They are not afraid to try and fail and try again.

I know for myself that my biggest learnings in life have come from my biggest fuck ups. Those fuck ups made me who I am today. They shaped and moulded me.

You can fail your way forwards and learn or you can stay the same. Although, staying the same is also a lesson in itself. You're still undergoing something. There's nothing wrong with that either.

A Higher Power Loves You

You always have free will. Even the Bible says God gave us free will. And that's the thing. Part of that free will is being able to make decisions which lead to learning about consequences. We're designed to make choices, possible mistakes and learn from it all.

I don't regret or take pity on myself for the trauma I suffered. It helped me discover my spiritual side, which has brought me so much inner peace. I have learnt there's a whole spiritual world out there that we can't normally see. It exists and it loves us. It's just pure love. We might not understand that. I have learnt to trust it really does love us all.

The higher realms want to help us so much. Everybody has a whole team of guides and ancestors in the spirit world that love them. They want to give support on our journeys through life. These divine beings want to serve our growth. Our evolution helps the world and universe. That ripple effect!

We're all doing this life thing alongside each other. Everyone and everything is always experiencing, individually and collectively. This includes spirit guides all the way up to the source or God. The universe itself is learning too. That's what people mean when they say you're the universe experiencing itself. We all are energy, we just take different forms. We're all the same substance, constantly shifting and vibrating through space.

We are interconnected with everything in the universe. Our guides want to step in and help where they can, but they can't sometimes unless you ask. This is because you always have free will. You don't have to ask them. You don't have to connect with them. You don't have to consciously be on a spiritual path either. That's still an experience. You also have a spirit. Hence your experience will always be spiritual. It does not have to be a conscious decision.

Have No Fear in the Dark

We as people like to label things as good or bad. I understand that's the duality of the universe.

It's said we live in a dualistic universe where there are positives and negatives. The Yin Yang symbol (depicted below) embodies this with its portrayals of the two contrasting energies in life. The light and the dark.

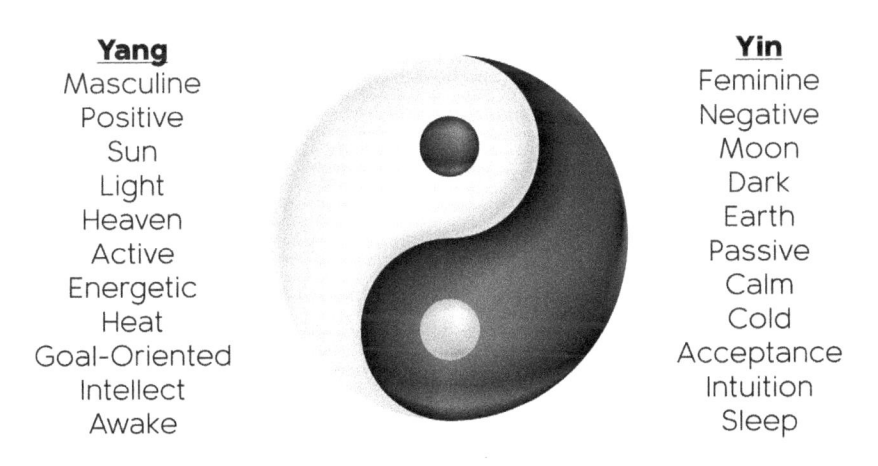

Yang	**Yin**
Masculine	Feminine
Positive	Negative
Sun	Moon
Light	Dark
Heaven	Earth
Active	Passive
Energetic	Calm
Heat	Cold
Goal-Oriented	Acceptance
Intellect	Intuition
Awake	Sleep

In this symbol, the larger section of black has a white circle and the larger section of white has a black circle. This represents how in every positive, there's a negative, and that in every negative there's a positive. It all comes down to perspective.

I prefer to use the terms dark and light rather than positive and negative. I think positive and negative comes with stigmas that things are good and bad. This is where I find we can slip up with our thinking.

Attaching good vs. bad, right vs. wrong labels can create stress within you. Whereas just observing it for what it is, without focusing on the negative, can reduce stress. Practicing mindfulness is a powerful way to detach from judgments, and be more neutral.

You can still recognise there are darker, denser energies and there are lighter, more free-flowing energies around us. However, be mindful of the meanings you attach when observing them.

Thoughts create our reality after all. Often what we focus on grows. If we focus on the negative, then more negatives will expand throughout our perspective and experience. Dark energies can be connected to the icky parts of existence, such as sickness and disease. However, that is all still spirit or the universe—it's just on a different spectrum. It's an experience.

I know this can be difficult to comprehend. It's not a mistake that darkness exists. It needs to be here. If it wasn't here, we wouldn't have the light to compare it to. How would we appreciate the goodness in life if we never knew suffering?

Without the dark, we wouldn't learn as effectively for we are motivated to change and grow when we are most uncomfortable. There would be nothing to compare the light with. There would be nothing better to strive towards. We would just be sitting in pure harmony and bliss. I know that's what we all would love. A lot of us would enjoy being in this constant oasis paradise. However, where is the progression? How boring would life be? Chaos and disorder must exist in order for harmony and balance to be appreciated. You cannot have one without the other.

Most of our significant growth occurs during unpleasant times, such as ones that cause pain and discomfort. An example would be when a little kid learns fire can burn them. Their mum might tell them not to touch it, yet they might not take that advice seriously.

The child learns very quickly not to touch it again once they get burnt though!

Creating Peace with Yourself and the Past

A healthy healing goal is practicing radical love and acceptance of where we are at, no matter where that is. It's great to want to move forwards and improve. It's important to remember that life is not meant to be taken as seriously as what our minds can trick us into believing at times. It's okay to poke fun at our "mistakes" and "shortcomings". Laughter is the best medicine after all. Don't get caught up being extra hard on yourself—nobody gains from you beating yourself up!

We aren't perfect, and that's what makes us perfect. No one is superior or inferior. We're just unique. We're experiencing different things based on our diverse past experiences.

Coming to this awareness has really helped me make peace with my past and previous choices I have made.

One instance this mindset especially benefitted me was with being abused. I just couldn't understand why this was happening to me. What did I do to deserve this? I felt like such a powerless victim.

Through healing, I really learned that life is not happening to me, life is happening for me. As fucked up as it sounds, being abused was for my greatest good. Don't get me wrong, that experience was absolutely scary. I wouldn't wish it upon anyone. I also used to beat myself up a lot and think dating my ex was a mistake, a complete waste.

I now see how much stronger and wiser it made me. He really taught me how to love and value myself. I was forced to after he broke me down that badly. Before him, I had spent a life resentful and desperate. I would self-sacrifice and please everyone at my own expense. I had no idea how to meet my own needs in a healthy way. I also saw the good in everyone and would be blind to any red flags.

Nowadays, I know what domestic violence looks like. I will never allow it to happen to me again. I actually know and understand what a boundary is! I fearlessly set them and in doing so, teach others how to treat me. I love myself and care for my needs more than I ever knew possible. I have learnt to feel so safe in my own company. I trust my decisions as I navigate life.

Through these realisations, I have been able to come to peace with that terrifying time in my life. I can still see the good that resulted from the awful amount of pain I lived through. There are no mistakes. That happened exactly how it needed to for me to personally evolve. It has blown me away how many women I have been able to support since overcoming domestic abuse. I would not have been able to if I had not already lived it myself.

The same thing can be said for the car accident and the terrible injuries I sustained. I firstly learnt an entirely new relationship with my body which I had never known before. I didn't even know what holistic health was prior. I also personally learnt how to overcome that level of trauma and disability. If I hadn't, I wouldn't be able to empathise with or help others going through similar health issues as I can today.

Everything happens for a reason, even if we can't fathom that reason. There's a bigger picture happening behind the scenes. We just have to learn to trust that life is happening for us, not to us.

Anytime in my life I thought I was making a mistake, I was actually being guided to a better path.

Sometimes we can feel like we are battling against life. All the directions you try to take are being blocked and it's uncomfortable. What I have learnt is in these instances, maybe we're being rejected for a reason. Maybe those directions are not for us. Maybe we're meant to be looking elsewhere. Maybe there's another perspective.

Anytime I thought I was making a mistake, I was actually gaining a deeper understanding of life, myself and others. We all have free will and our free will leads us to consequences. Sometimes we have to go through difficulties and challenges in order to strengthen our character.

Life often gives us not what we want, but what we need. What we need is usually not only for our own highest good—but also for the greater good of the planet.

Healing Yourself

The biggest takeaway I can give from this book is that learning, healing, and developing, all come down to us as individuals. We can be helped and supported. At the end of the day, nobody is coming to fix or save us. We have to be responsible for our own well-being. Healing is not about forcing other people around us to change. It involves holding ourselves accountable.

Healing is about yourself. How can you be better than the person you were yesterday? A week ago? A year ago? This isn't a race or competition against others. This is your personal progress. There's no rush.

Occasionally you don't think you're getting anywhere. It's as if you're going around in circles. Healing is not linear. It really is the saying—fall down seven times, stand up eight or three steps forward, two steps back.

Trust that where you're at is never a mistake. It's the journey of life, the experience, the human condition. It isn't meant to be taken as seriously as we think. We're all on a journey. Yet we are travelling over time, the universe, on this space rock that gives us so much life. Whilst we're roaming through life, our soul is learning. We as a collective consciousness are expanding from what is experienced. You've just got to follow where your heart takes you. It can be that simple.

You might fall out of balance and that's okay. It's just another experience. Becoming more aware and then trying to come back into that balance takes practice. That is all it is. It's just a path of existing and undergoing situations that teach you more about yourself, others and life.

Although I say there are no mistakes, that doesn't mean there aren't consequences. People usually refer to this concept as karma. What you give is what you get. For example, if you're out in life hurting people, it will catch up to you. It's not a punishment. You aren't a victim of life. It's more of an experience that aims at helping you grow as a person. What you've been giving out is usually what you attract so it's only fair to be on the receiving end. Or you may not. This is where if it doesn't catch up to you in this life, it probably will in a future lifetime. For every action, there's an opposite reaction. A balancing act. Throughout the entire universe.

You might say that God and spirituality aren't real.

That's cool. I completely understand and accept that being your view. I'm not here to convert or shove religions or spiritual beliefs on people. I'm just sharing the perspective that has helped me overcome past traumatic experiences. I now feel the most peace and fulfilment that I ever have in my life.

You might say that bad people are evil. Don't make excuses for them.

I agree. I'm not condoning bad behaviour. What I'm saying is these people are also playing their role. Maybe their soul needs to experience and exist in lots of darkness in order to grow the most in this lifetime. I know it can be a difficult concept to wrap your head around, but again, you don't have to take it on board just because I've written a book.

Some mistakes can be terrible. You can't say there aren't any.

I understand that's your perspective and your judgment. Why label something as good versus bad? Maybe it is just a neutral event. If every positive has a negative and every negative has a positive surely they can cancel one another out and become neutral. It's just what needs to be experienced and learnt about. There's always a hero and a villain in every story—it just depends on who the narrator is. I don't expect this to be widely understood. I do ask you to try to invite a more open perspective in and see what shifts occur with this understanding in mind.

Accepting Mistakes

Practice forgiving yourself for the past. You didn't know then what you know now. It's okay. Forgive yourself for the future too whilst you're at it. Mistakes are an inevitable part of life. There's no use comparing yourself to other people, we're all different and works in progress.

I like to write forgiveness letters to myself and others from my past, expressing my thoughts and feelings.

Gentle self-talk to reassure yourself or simply having a laugh about it assists if you catch yourself stewing on what should or could have been.

I also recommend writing a list of the biggest mistakes that you think you've made in life. Then next to them, write what you learned from these mistakes and see what comes up. Also see if you can brainstorm how you could possibly use this mistake to help other people, using your strengths and skills. Experiences are gifts and sharing wisdom gained from them can help others.

Summary

If you want change, do something differently. Staying the same will normally only give you more of what you've already gotten. You may think you're too far gone, too broken, too much. If you think this, please know that you're someone whose purpose is even more powerful than you realise.

We gain most of our wisdom from mistakes and hard experiences. It's never too late. You're never too fucked up.

You can start anywhere. There's always going to be people doing better than you. Just as there will always be people doing worse than you. Start somewhere by trying something you haven't done before.

If you feel called to help others, there's always going to be someone who is a little bit behind where you're at and you have knowledge that will help them. Whilst everyone is always a student of life, everyone is also a teacher.

Please understand your insight and experiences are important and needed. They never were mistakes and it's okay to make them. They are stories to be shared.

We have gifts inside of us, including knowledge, and there are people out there waiting to connect with it. Whether you realise it or not, you can tap into that power. Do you want to tap into those gifts? You don't have to. Though if you feel drawn to it, go for it. Just start somewhere—the worst that can happen is you give up and return to where you were before.

Despite how many mistakes you may believe you have made, you always have something to offer. Whether you realise it or not, your existence is important in this world and it's needed.

All you need to do is be yourself.

That's why I called my business Beecoming You, asides from loving bumble bees. I believe all we need to do is be ourselves, whatever that may mean. I think that practicing acceptance of the past whilst also striving to fearlessly build a better future is a key part of being able to heal and overcome trauma.

Afterword

Congratulations and thank you for getting to the end! I have the utmost gratitude for you taking the time to read my life's story so far. Whilst we are all unique, we are all here sharing the breath of life. We don't all have to agree, for we are altogether experiencing life differently—past, present, and future. Thank you for giving the care and time from your own life to read mine.

Writing this book ended up taking longer than originally planned. I was hit with fears about sharing my story and doubting if it was even worth telling.

Meanwhile, I felt like a fraud as I faced being present when someone violently hurt themselves, and having people in my life betray me around the time of my manuscript's deadline. My uncle also passed away suddenly not long after I had my arm operated on, so I went through another injury recovery journey.

I found myself in despair, running from telling my story. What I realise now is that is okay. There was no mistake in it.

I was writing a book on trauma, after all. In the extra months this book took me to write, I was thrown pretty heavy challenges. I was given a chance to truly practice what I'm preaching. I applied the knowledge and therapies this book includes and I have successfully bounced back from these challenges even lighter, brighter and more confident than I was before.

Finally, I suggest trying to not close yourself off to the possibilities that life presents. Try not to let the past define you—you have the ability to define the future based on your choices today. It's never too late. It's possible to change! Opportunity is everywhere.

You can overcome obstacles. Learn to let go of the idea that you're stuck and helpless. Where there's a will, there's a way. Solutions are possible. Lead with love over fear. Love for life, love for others, and love for yourself. Even if you can only find one thing you love about life, others, or yourself. You never know, appreciating that one thing may lead you to appreciate more.

About the Author

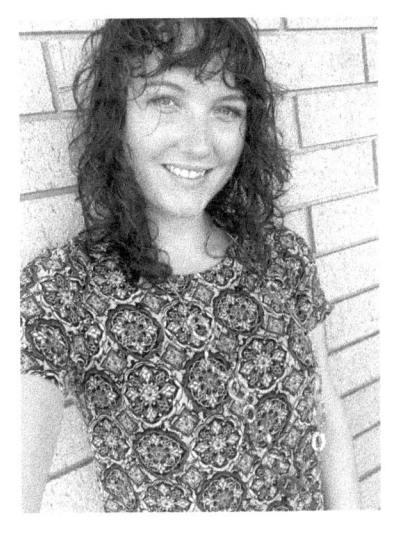

Rachie grew up in the Rockingham and Mandurah regions of Western Australia. She enjoys spending her time painting, at the beach, gardening and with loved ones. During her colourful life, involving domestic violence and a major car accident, she has learnt how to bounce back and triumph over trauma.

Rach's curious nature has also led her to become qualified with a BA in psychology with minors in developmental and health psychology, colour mirrors therapy, Reiki, crystal, metaphysical and animal healing.

After experiencing struggles with her mental health and a sense of belonging from a young age, Rach was taken on a journey of self-discovery that led to a deeper understanding of others and life. Her hopes for the future are to be able to assist others in learning to help themselves using her knowledge and skills.

All in all, Rachie wishes to help people reconnect with the magic and beauty that exists in life.

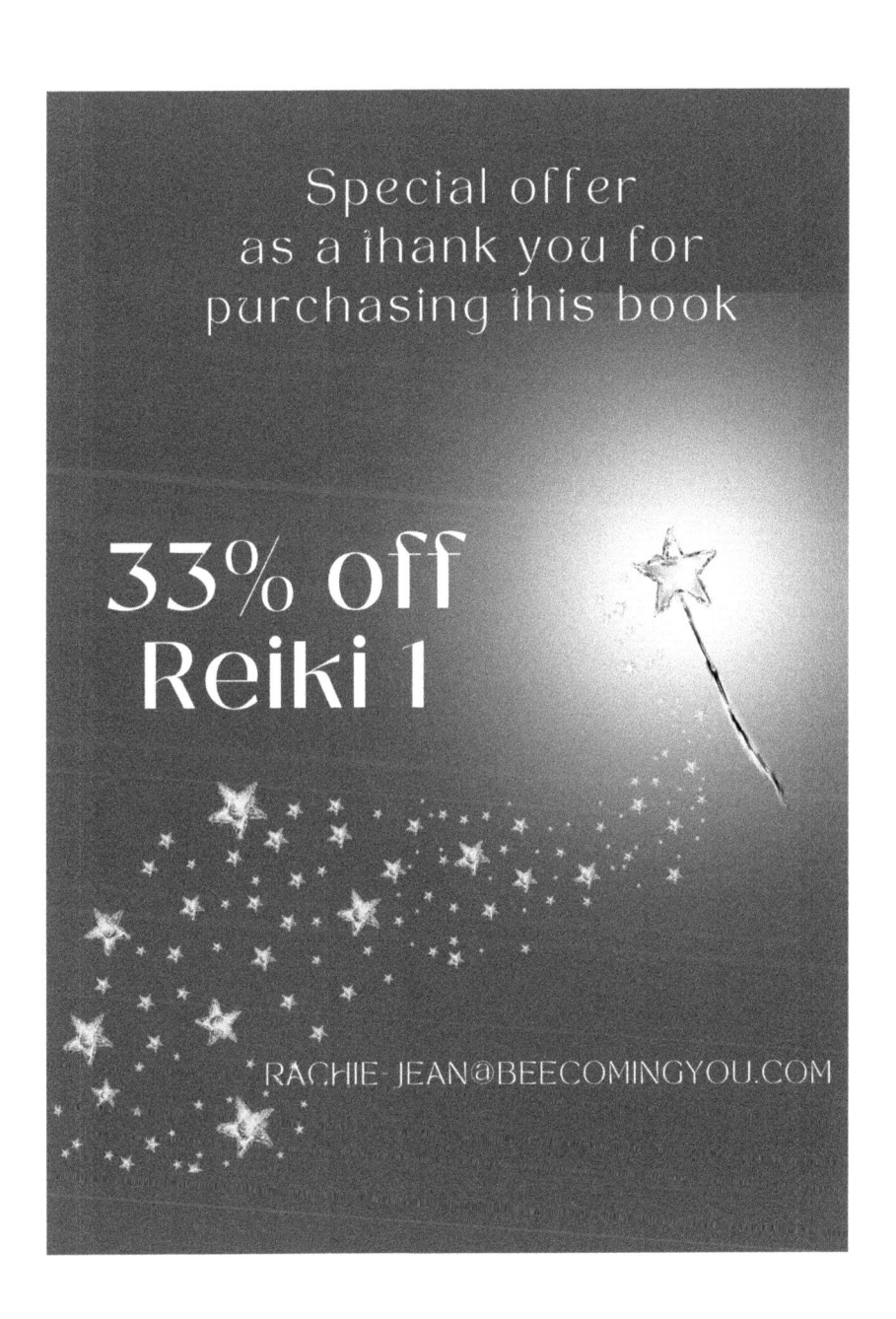

Special offer
as a thank you for
purchasing this book

33% off
Reiki 1

RACHIE-JEAN@BEECOMINGYOU.COM

References

[1] Gustafson, C. "Bruce Lipton, Phd: The Jump from Cell Culture to Consciousness." *Integrative Medicine (Encinitas, Calif.)*, U.S. National Library of Medicine, pubmed.ncbi.nlm.nih.gov/30936816/.

[2] Freud, Sigmund. *The Question of Lay Analysis; an Introduction to Psychoanalysis*. Norton, 1950.

[3] Northrup, Christiane. *Dodging Energy Vampires: An Empath's Guide to Evading Relationships That Drain You and Restoring Your Health and Power*. Hay House, 2018.

[4] Connolly, Korani, and Melissie Jolly. *The Wisdom of Colour Mirrors*. Lightning Source, 2019.

[5] Jain, Felipe A., et al. "Critical Analysis of the Efficacy of Meditation Therapies for Acute and Subacute Phase Treatment of Depressive Disorders: A Systematic Review." *Psychosomatics*, vol. 56, no. 2, 22 Oct. 2014, pp. 140–152, doi:10.1016/j.psym.2014.10.007.

Further Testimonials

"I have had the pleasure of knowing Rachie from our earlier years of bartending before the accident. I followed her journey as she bravely and patiently allowed herself the time, space and grace to heal from the accident. Very true to her Taurean nature, she took the slow and steady path of healing. Not only her physical injuries but the energetic and emotional ones that we sometimes encounter through just being a human on Earth. It hasn't appeared to be the easiest road but through it all, she was wholeheartedly herself. Kind, light-hearted, incredibly brave and resilient. The light was always there within her, shining bright and that is such a testament to her beautiful inner strength and courage. We both went on separate paths for most of her healing journey, as I was on a healing journey myself. Though somehow, our paths have crossed again years later, and I am lucky to call Rachie a dear friend now. I have experienced her powerful healing energy through receiving Reiki from her or by accessing her divine guidance through our conversations and card-pulling sessions. It's remarkable the life she has already experienced at such a young age and the wisdom she has accumulated because of it. To then put that experience and wisdom into her book for us to read, well, we are truly in for a treat."

– **Agi Szabo**

"Recently while at work, I suffered a serious tear to my calf muscle. This immediately left me unable to walk or work.

After the initial visit to the emergency department, I was told the injury would see me off work for 4-6 weeks and I would need extensive physio and rehabilitation for that to happen.

Although I'd never tried before, or knew anything about Reiki, when Rachael suggested it might be really helpful, I didn't hesitate.

The result was truly unbelievable, I was back at work on full duties after 2 weeks. The physiotherapist put me through the full range of return-to-work exercises after only my second of 10 scheduled appointments, she couldn't believe how quickly I recovered.

Thank you, Rachael. What you did was amazing."

– **Marty Tabak**

"I met Rachael just months before she got into her accident so I am mostly familiar with 'after' Rachael. We bonded while I visited her in the hospital and even back then I was astounded by her strength. She made it sound like the crash was not that serious and she was fine. Upon catching up with her, she would just very calmly explain how she was in horrible pain and that she had to have another operation. Her words were silent, her actions spoke louder and she was caught in a downward spiral, making dangerous decisions and going crazy with mental and physical pain. And then it just stopped. Rachael found a strength within herself to break the spiral and to live and accept the cards destiny has dealt her. She is a beautiful soul, has been misunderstood by many and has overcome hardships many her age never have to experience. I am proud to be able to call her my friend."

– **Jana Unger**

Further Testimonials

"When I first met Rachael, I loved her vibrant spirit, but a deep tiredness permeated her visions of the future. At a young age, she'd already endured so much physical and mental trauma. Rach's healing journey found her exploring both conventional and alternative therapies, reigniting her passion for life and finding her purpose in helping others."

– Natalie Goddard

Notes

From Trauma to Triumph

Notes

From Trauma to Triumph

Notes